milk soaps

Making Milk-Enriched Soaps
from Goat to Almond

• • • —— • —— • •

ANNE-MARIE FAIOLA

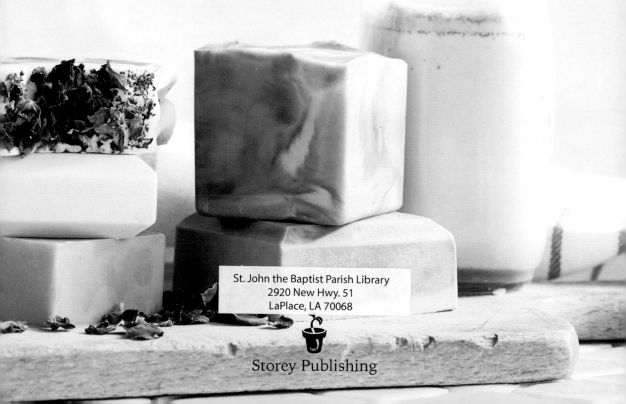

Storey Publishing

The mission of Storey Publishing is to serve our customers by publishing practical information that encourages personal independence in harmony with the environment.

Edited by Deborah Balmuth and Lisa H. Hiley
Art direction and book design by Michaela Jebb
Text production by Jennifer Jepson Smith
Indexed by Nancy D. Wood

Cover photography by © Charity Burggraaf, except back, author by Amanda Kerzman and back, top left by © Mariemlulu/iStock.com
Interior photography by © Charity Burggraaf, except © FotografiaBasica/Getty Images, 13 top right; Mars Vilaubi, 52, 76, 106, 136, 170, 252; © MilaDrumeva/iStock.com, 5
Photo styling by Mandy Kehoe
How-to diagrams by Ilona Sherratt

Storey Publishing
210 MASS MoCA Way
North Adams, MA 01247
storey.com

Printed in China by Printplus Ltd.
10 9 8 7 6 5 4 3 2 1

LIBRARY OF CONGRESS CATALOGING-IN-PUBLICATION DATA

Names: Faiola, Anne-Marie, author.
Title: Milk soaps : 35 skin-nourishing recipes for making milk-enriched soaps, from goat to almond / by Anne-Marie Faiola.
Description: North Adams, MA : Storey Publishing, [2019] | Includes index.
Identifiers: LCCN 2018044865 (print) | LCCN 2018045045 (ebook) | ISBN 9781635860498 (ebook) | ISBN 9781635860481 (hardcover with concealed wire-o : alk. paper)
Subjects: LCSH: Soap.
Classification: LCC TP991 (ebook) | LCC TP991 .F278 2019 (print) | DDC 668/.12—dc23
LC record available at https://lccn.loc.gov/2018044865

Be sure to read all the instructions thoroughly before undertaking any of the projects in this book and follow all the safety guidelines.

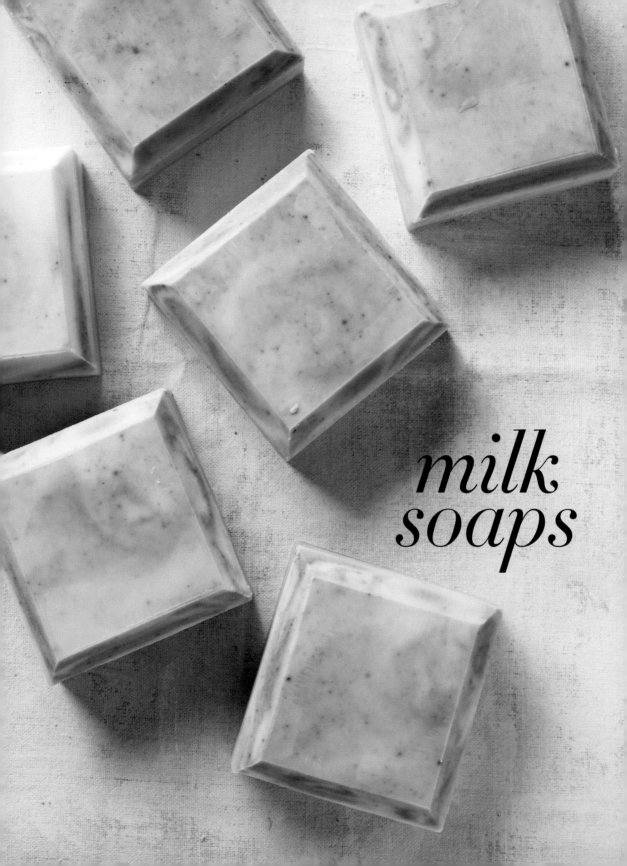

milk soaps

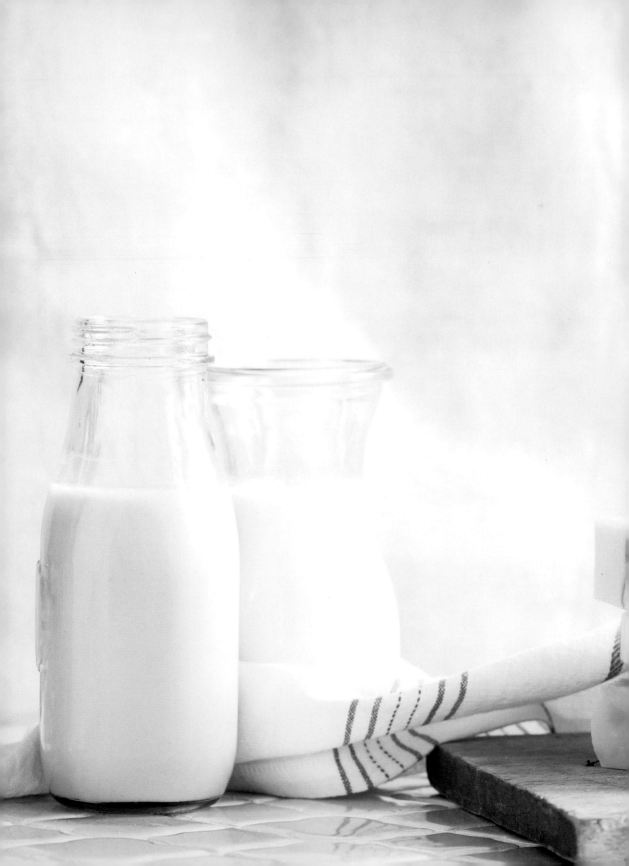

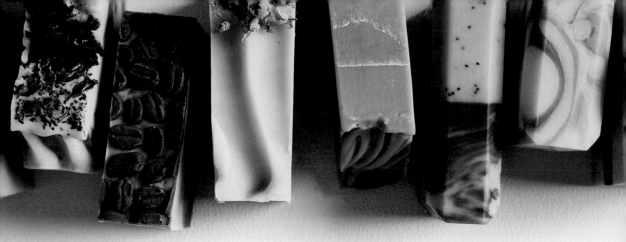

Contents

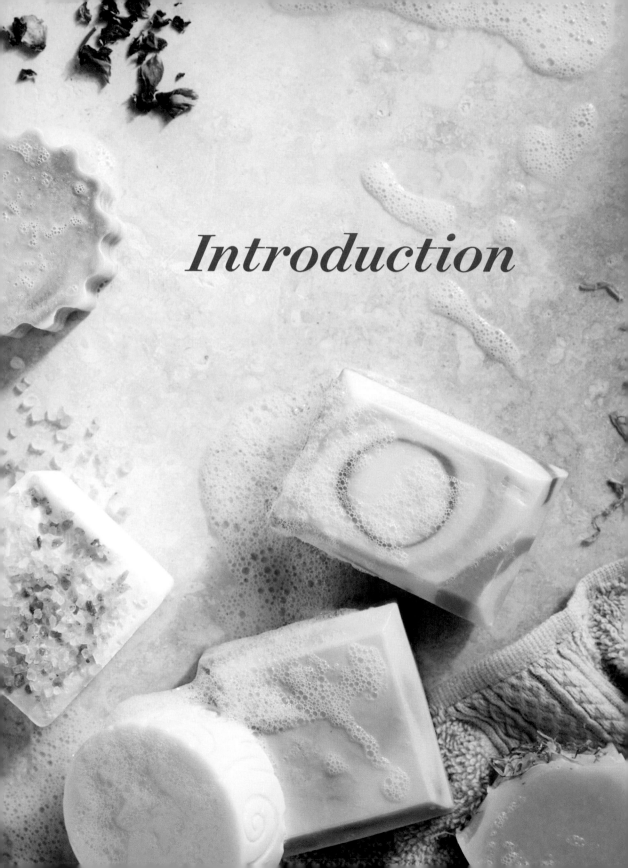

Introduction

"Handmade is bestmade" is a tagline we frequently use at Bramble Berry. It's true for almost everything. Think of artisanal cheeses and breads — yum, right? Handmade shrubs and bitters? Amazing. The same goes for handmade soap — it's just better. It feels better, looks and smells better, and performs better. You can choose the most skin-loving, gentle, and conditioning ingredients when you're crafting with purpose, and the end result shows it.

Handmade soap may not be the cheapest choice (it's hard to compete with pressed sodium lauryl sulfate on price), but you won't have to slather on lotions or creams after using it because it doesn't strip your skin of natural oils. Synthetic lathering agents do provide lather and high cleansing ability, but those copious bubbles dissolve essential skin oils as they wipe clean the ravages of the day. Handmade soap simply feels better on the skin; it pampers as it cleans.

Another reason handmade is bestmade is because you control the colors and the fragrance. Want your soap to match your bathroom or smell like your grandma's garden? Are you planning a bridal shower and want to follow the color theme of the wedding? Done, done, and done! The process of soapmaking is one of transformation: transforming oils into something new, useful, and beautiful. Having a creative outlet is essential in all of our lives, and soapmaking provides a beautiful way to express yourself.

I've been making soap by hand since I was a teenager. I remember rendering my own tallow, trying to decode chemistry textbooks, and wondering why I couldn't use Drāno to make soap. My first five batches failed. I had to figure out how to dispose of caustic failed soap, but it was a thrill to give away my first successful batches, molded in Rubbermaid containers, chopped up with a knife, and wrapped in plastic wrap. At age 17, shaking like a leaf, I walked into a local store with a basket of my wares, hoping to sell my soap. I was rejected. The bars weren't uniform enough. I returned a month later with a signature mold style and shape that would later become Bramble Berry's first custom mold. I landed the account. After that I was hooked.

The idea that I could create, control my ingredients, be an alchemical artist, and make money was magical. Through the lens of soapmaking, science felt supremely useful. At the time there were no soapmaking books, save one that utilized Crisco for most of its recipes. That's one of the reasons I was inspired to write my first two books, *Soap Crafting* and *Pure Soapmaking*. I wanted to create the books I wished had been around when I started my journey into soapmaking.

With this book, I'm taking that journey to the world of milk-enriched soapmaking. These recipes are designed to appeal to a wide variety of soapers — fans of all-natural products, people who prefer palm-free soaps, casual and expert soapers alike. Each recipe that utilizes synthetic ingredients for design purposes offers all-natural alternatives that will bring you similar results. Each recipe has been created by an expert soapmaker and tested multiple times by brand-new soapers in order to account for every variable, so whether this is your first batch with cold-process soap or milk soap or your hundredth, you'll get consistent results every time. Handmade is bestmade, and I'm so happy you've chosen to take this journey with me.

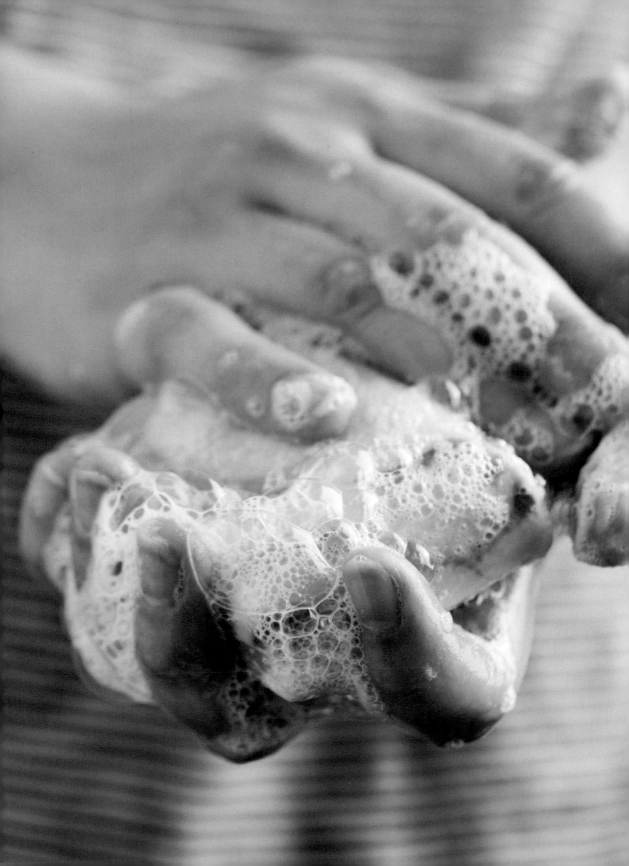

CHAPTER ONE

Why Make Soap with Milk?

Most soaps are made with water, but you can use any liquid that has a pH above 6: milk, tea, even beer and wine. So why an entire book dedicated to making soap with milk? Well, it's kind of like drinking hot chocolate made with milk instead of hot chocolate made with water.

Milk soap is creamier and more luscious than soap made with water. The lather is more dense. The foam is more fine and silkier. Milk soaps have the same cleansing power, but milk's natural oils and acids pump up the skin-loving moisture quotient and aid in skin renewal.

Animal-based milks contain a small amount of lactic acid, which acts as a gentle exfoliant. As it cleanses, it helps remove dead skin cells to reveal smoother skin. Animal-based milks also have naturally occurring amino acids and a host of skin-loving vitamins. When making soap, the more fat you have in the milk, the more those delightful lipids interact with the glycerin and nourishing oils in the recipe to create a treat for your skin. I like to soap with full-fat milk, but you can use any version in these recipes.

Plant-based milks work equally well (see page 8). While these recipes have been formulated with specific milks, you can substitute any milk for the one called for in any recipe.

Using Mammal Milks

Some popular milks to make soap with include the following.

Cow's Milk

Cow's milk is the most readily available animal milk, though milk from other animals is increasingly easy to locate, depending on where you live. The fat molecules in cow's milk are larger than in other animal milks, which is why some lactose-intolerant individuals can drink goat's milk instead. In soap, the size of fat molecules does not have much bearing on the final product.

Cow's milk is slightly higher in sugar than goat's milk, leading to larger, creamier bubbles in the final product. It is higher in vitamin B_{12} and vitamin D, as well as folate and selenium, than goat's and sheep's milk. The vitamins and selenium are especially skin-loving antioxidants that help repair free-radical damage. Folate (also known as vitamin B_9) is important for skin cell renewal and growth.

Goat's Milk

Goat's milk soap is one of the best-known types of handmade soap. It is popular because of its nourishing properties. Goat's milk is full of nourishing vitamins helpful to skin, like A, B_1, B_6, B_{12}, C, D, and E. It is also high in naturally occurring enzymes and proteins. Goat's milk has a reputation for having natural antimicrobial properties and for being good for acne.

You'll also see claims that goat's milk soap is best for difficult skin conditions such as psoriasis and eczema because goat's milk soap contains caprylic acid. Caprylic acid is naturally found in goat's milk, though it's more commonly associated with coconut oil and liquid glycerin.

Sour Milk?

Milk spoils on your counter. Why doesn't it spoil in soap? The high pH of the soap mixture ensures that the bacteria that spoils milk are fully neutralized in the soapmaking process. The richness the milk gives the soap is still present in the final bar.

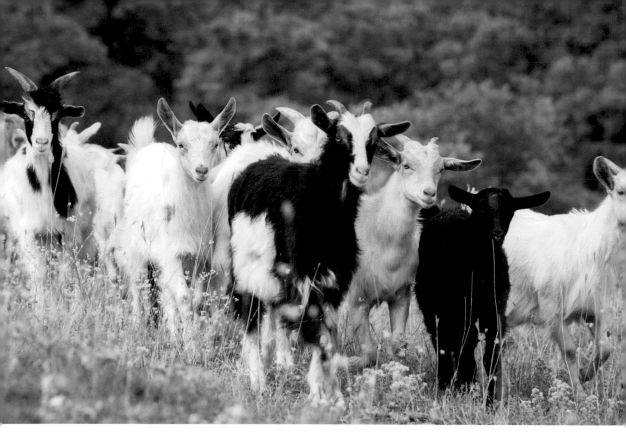

It adds to the silkiness of goat's milk soap, bumps up the antioxidants, and is a fantastic emollient and moisturizing agent.

Many believe that goat's milk's medium-chain fatty acids (there's caprylic acid at work again!) help goat's milk penetrate the first layer of (mostly dead) skin to encourage effective movement and deposition of the fat-soluble vitamins A, E, and K. Vitamins A and E are natural antioxidants, which means they can neutralize free radicals before they can damage your skin. (Free radicals are highly reactive atoms or molecules that cause all sorts of havoc in the body.)

Dairy goat's milk varies in percentage of fat depending on the type of goat. For example, Nigerian dairy goats produce more cream than any other dairy breed. Goat's milk is not readily available in most supermarkets, so you will have to buy it directly from a farmer or specialty grocery store. That generally means you will be making soap with raw milk that has not been pasteurized or homogenized.

Other Mammal Milks

Other mammal milks include sheep's milk, camel's milk, and donkey's milk. Sheep's milk is excellent for soapmaking because it is much whiter than other animal milks. Sheep's milk is high in fat and conjugated linoleic acid, which makes it an excellent emollient and moisturizer. It has very small fat globules and therefore is naturally homogenized. Typically, sheep's milk is only available directly from a farmer.

Camel's milk is popular with the paleo community because it is casein-free and contains naturally occurring omega-3 fatty acids. Like sheep's milk, it is naturally homogenized, which means it can be frozen and thawed without changing its consistency. Because of its popularity with this crowd, it can be purchased in some stores or via mail order. It has a high amount of vitamins and minerals and is three times higher in vitamin C than cow's milk. It also has a high level of vitamin B compared to other animal milks. One downside to camel's milk is its expense: camels are far rarer in North America than cows, and they produce less milk.

If you are lucky enough to come across donkey's milk, definitely make soap with it. Although it's extremely low in fat, it is loaded with protein and lactose. It also contains essential amino acids, bioactive enzymes and coenzymes, and four times more vitamin C than cow's milk.

Using Plant Milks

Plant-based milks are a fantastic alternative to mammal milks in making soap. While they don't provide the same qualities, they do provide an option for those who don't use dairy products. They also have a certain amount of label cachet and a strong marketing appeal. A nut- or grain-based milk adds the same vitamins, minerals, and nutrients to soap that it offers nutritionally. For example, oat milk contains vitamins A, B, and E, all strong antioxidants. Almond milk is high in vitamin E and also contains magnesium, which helps manage skin oiliness.

Coconut Milk

Coconut milk increases lather and adds conditioning properties to soap by supplying fatty acids. Half of the fatty acids in coconut milk is lauric acid, which many believe to be antimicrobial. And coconut milk soap does not discolor as much as goat's milk soap, giving you more flexibility with color options. When you are shopping for coconut milk, look for brands without guar gum, a thickener and retarder of ice crystals. Two brands that typically do not contain guar gum are Goya and Roland.

Nut Milks

Nut milks can be made from any raw, unsalted, and unshelled nut. The more common nuts used to make milk are almonds, cashews, peanuts, and hazelnuts. For soapmaking, it's best to make your own nut milk to ensure that it's free of additives. If you do use a store-bought nut milk, choose an unflavored one with the fewest ingredients and no added sugar. Sugars heat up in the soapmaking process, which can scorch your soap and lead to spillover in the molds or soap splitting as it hardens.

Yes, You Can Use Breast Milk

Believe it or not, people do use human breast milk to make soap. It is higher in fat than cow's or goat's milk. It also contains lots of sugar and vitamins A, (retinol), C, D, and E. If soapmaking with breast milk, follow the basic instructions for other mammal milks (freeze the milk, add the sodium hydroxide to it slowly, and keep the superfat at 10 percent or below).

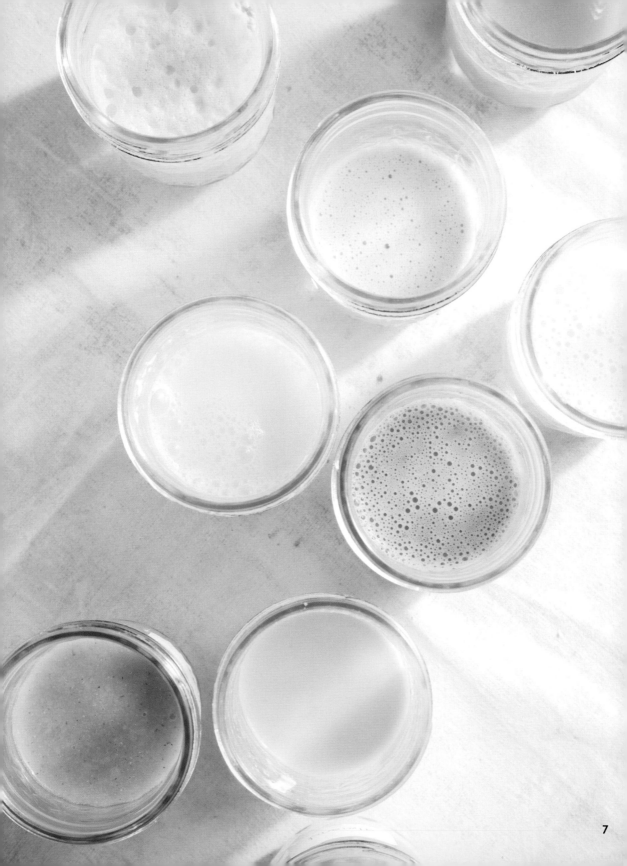

How to Make Nut, Grain, and Seed Milks

Making nut milk is simple, but it takes advance planning. The basic process is to soak a quantity of raw nuts in at least twice as much water for one or two days, then blend them with water and strain the resulting liquid. Some seeds, such as flax, absorb quite a lot of water and must be soaked in 6 cups of water before blending them (no straining required).

This recipe yields about 2 cups (473 mL) of nut milk.

- 1 cup (237 mL) raw nuts
- 2–4 cups (472–946 mL) distilled water for soaking
- 3 cups (709 mL) distilled water for blending
- Sieve or colander
- Cheesecloth, jelly bag, strainer, or nut milk bag
- Ice cube trays

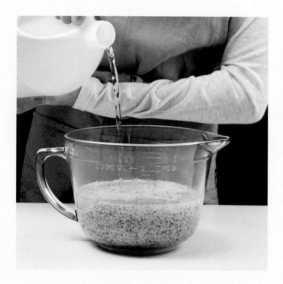 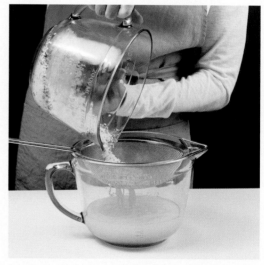

1 Place the nuts in a container with enough distilled water to cover them by 2 inches. Let them soak overnight in the refrigerator. After 24 hours, the nuts should have taken up a lot of the water and will feel a bit squishy. If you want a creamier milk, soak them for another day.

2 When the nuts have soaked to your liking, pour them into a colander and rinse until the water runs clear. (Tap water is fine for rinsing.) Discard the soaking water.

If the nuts have skins (like almonds or hazelnuts), you might want to peel them. This can take some time, but it makes blending and straining easier and produces a cleaner milk.

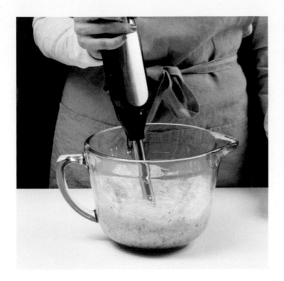

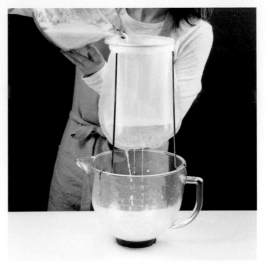

3 Place the nuts and distilled water in a blender and blend on high for 2 or 3 minutes, or until they are fully blended. Alternatively, use a stick blender, making sure that the nuts are finely ground. The mixture should be white.

4 Strain the mixture through a sieve to remove the largest particles. Strain a second time through cheesecloth, a jelly strainer, or a nut milk bag.

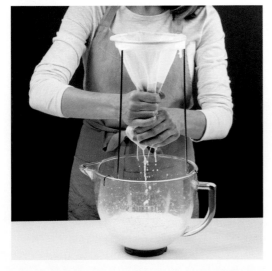

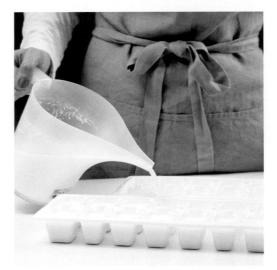

5 Squeeze as much milk from the pulp as possible.

6 The milk can be stored in the refrigerator for up to 4 days (if it separates, just shake it up again). Or pour the milk into ice cube trays in 1-ounce (28 g) portions and freeze.

Using Leftover Nut Pulp

You can dehydrate the leftover pulp into flour by following these steps and use it as an exfoliant for soaps or other skin-care products. If you used regular kitchen equipment (not your soap-making stick blender), you can add the flour to baked goods.

1   Heat the oven to its lowest setting. Line a cookie sheet with parchment paper. (Or use a dehydrator with fruit leather mats.)

2   Spread the pulp out evenly on the cookie sheet and bake until dry and crumbly. This could take several hours, depending on how moist the pulp is.

3   Let the dried pulp cool, then blend into a powder in a blender or with a stick blender. The finer the powder, the gentler its exfoliation action in soaps or scrubs.

Rice Milk

Rice milk is another ingredient prized for its skin-loving properties. Rice milk is naturally sweeter than many nut milks, giving the soap lots of bubbles and lather. It is made by pressing cooked rice through a mill and straining out the pressed grains. You can make it at home by boiling 1 cup of rice in 4 cups of water, blending it, and straining the mixture, a process similar to making nut milks. You can also buy rice milk; just stay away from additives that might compromise your recipe.

Oat Milk

Oat milk is a popular alternative-milk option, with enormous label appeal. It is full of vitamins A, B, C, D, and E, all strong antioxidants that help protect skin against harmful free radicals. A low-cost product, it produces smooth, rich, and creamy soap. The milk itself is not as liquid as other milks; in fact, it's rather sticky and gooey. The stickiness is reduced if it's made with steel-cut oats. The pulp takes longer to dry than other grain or nut pulp.

Oat milk reacts poorly with lye, so it's best added at trace (see page 30) to prevent it from congealing.

To make oat milk, follow the directions for making nut milk, but rinse and drain the oats before soaking them. Use 1 cup (237 mL) steel-cut oats per 3 cups (709 ml) distilled water. Oat milk freezes well.

Seed Milks

Many seed-based milks, such as hempseed or pumpkin seed, are made in the same way as nut milks, by soaking the seeds overnight and then blending them with water. Flaxseeds, however, turn gelatinous in liquid, so soak each cup (237 mL) of seeds in 6 cups (1,419 mL) of distilled water.

The resulting mixture is too thick to strain, so skip that step and blend each cup of the soaked seeds with an additional 3 cups of distilled water. This produces a thick, gelatinous milk that soaps well when added 30 percent at trace. As with nut milks, you can freeze seed milks to store them; most recipes call for thawing before adding them.

Special Techniques for Working with Milk

There are a couple ways to incorporate milk into soap, and the method you choose can dramatically affect the initial scent and final color of the bars. Milk is full of natural sugars, proteins, vitamins, and minerals. To make caramel for eating (yum), you heat milk and butter or cream until it (you guessed it!) caramelizes.

In soapmaking, the sugars in the milk caramelize and mix with the high-pH sodium hydroxide, creating a foul smell. All freshly cut and freshly unmolded milk soaps, no matter which method of handling used, smell bad. This smell goes away after about 10 days, leaving just the scent of the fragrance or essential oil. Caramelization also, depending on temperatures used, gives soap its color, ranging from ivory to brown.

Most of the recipes in this book call for frozen milk, not liquid. It's recommended that you freeze the milk before mixing it with lye to prevent the mixture from overheating, which scorches the milk, discoloring it and making it smell awful. A few recipes call for adding liquid milk at trace (once the batter is mixed) rather than adding to the lye mixture. Frozen milk can be thawed for use in these recipes.

Using Milk at 100 Percent

A 100 percent milk soap is created when you substitute 100 percent of the water in a recipe for some form of milk. While easy to formulate, the method has some drawbacks. Because the lye directly contacts the milk, the milk proteins are prone to scorching. Using the frozen milk

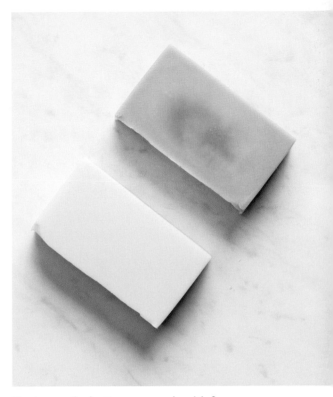

The bar on the bottom was made with frozen milk; the one on the top with lye added directly to liquid milk.

method described on page 12 helps reduce the scorching.

Milk can contain up to 40 percent fat. Since soapmaking requires one lye molecule for every fat molecule, up to 60 percent of the liquid you add to the recipe will not have a lye partner to pair up with. For this reason, when using 100 percent milk, some soapers prefer to soap at a lower superfat than a soap made with water. (For more on the science of soaping and a description of cold-process soapmaking, see chapter 2.)

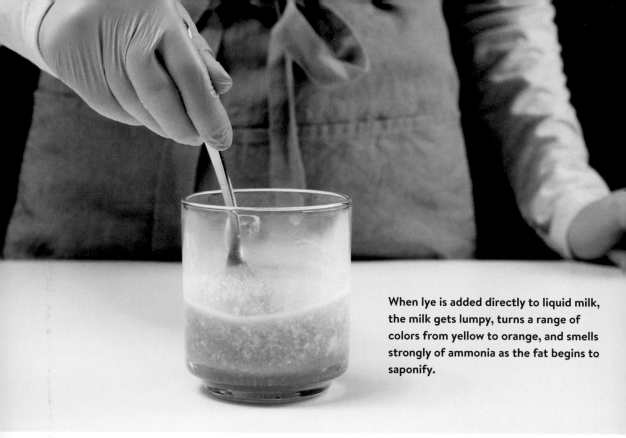

When lye is added directly to liquid milk, the milk gets lumpy, turns a range of colors from yellow to orange, and smells strongly of ammonia as the fat begins to saponify.

The Frozen Milk Method

Milk proteins scorch when exposed to heat; by freezing the milk, you lower the temperature of the entire process and slow down the reaction with the lye. Working with very cold milk also helps decrease the distinctive ammonia smell during the soapmaking process, and it gives your soap a more neutral final color, an ivory or light tan.

This technique takes a bit longer because you add the lye a tablespoon (15 mL) at a time, stirring constantly as the milk melts. As the lye reacts with the milk's fat molecules, the mixture may turn yellow or orange and start to smell bad. It may also turn lumpy as the lye partners up with the milk fat.

Continue adding the lye slowly to help prevent scorching, stirring constantly. Let the mixture sit for 20 to 30 minutes to ensure that all the lye particles are fully dissolved, then give it one final stir before you proceed with the recipe.

If the lye doesn't appear to be fully dissolved, let it sit longer and stir, stir, stir before pouring the lye-milk mixture through a fine-mesh strainer to add it to the oils to ensure no lye flakes make it into the soap.

Note: Frozen milk can be stored in the freezer for up to a year. Freeze milk in ice cube trays and store in labeled freezer bags.

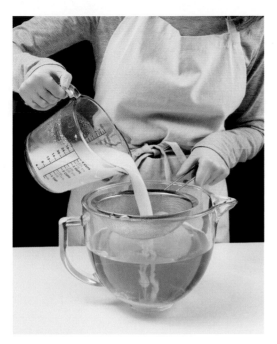

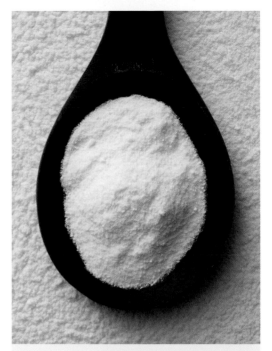

Always add frozen milk–lye mixture to the oils by pouring it through a fine-mesh strainer. Use a spoon or spatula to gently stir any residue through the holes.

Using Powdered Milk

All of these recipes can be made with any type of mammal milk, and that includes powdered products. Just make the powdered milk according to the instructions and measure out the required amount for the recipe. As with all commercial products, choose a brand that has the least number of additives possible.

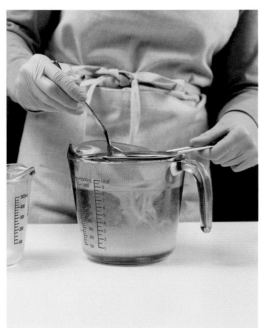

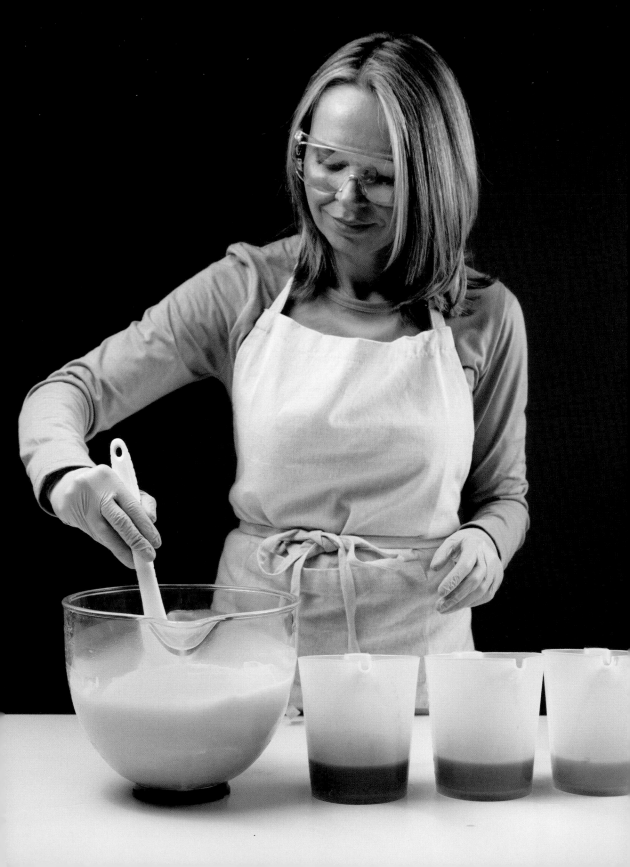

CHAPTER TWO

The Soapmaking
Process

• • • —————— • —————— • • •

Soapmaking is pure chemistry. The mixture of a high-pH substance (sodium hydroxide, or lye) and various oils (vegetable- or animal-based), when balanced correctly, turns into soap. At its simplest, the chemical formula is lye + oil = soap. But the lye needs a carrier in order to mix with the oil, so the formula is actually (lye + carrier liquid) + oil = soap. The recipes in this book use mammal and nut milks combined with water as the carrier liquid.

Making soap from scratch is often called *cold-process soapmaking* because the chemical reaction between the lye and the carrier liquid heats the mixture up so rapidly that no outside heat source is needed to melt the oils. Modern-day soapmakers typically do use a microwave or stove to melt oils and butters to ensure a consistent recipe, but technically, it's not needed. *Never* reheat lye-water or a mixed soap batter.

Calculating the SAP Value

The process by which the lye and the oils bond to create a new substance is called *saponification*. Each oil requires a different ratio of sodium hydroxide to turn into soap. The ratio of lye needed for a particular oil is its *saponification value* (or SAP *value*). The SAP value multiplied by the ounces of oil in a given recipe tells you how much lye is needed. The math needed to create a perfectly balanced soap is simple, if sometimes cumbersome.

Here's an example: How much lye is needed to make soap with 100 ounces (2.8 kg) of coconut oil? The SAP value of coconut oil is 0.178, so the math looks like this:

SAP value (0.178) × amount of oil (100 ounces/ 2.8 kg) = 17.8 ounces (504 g) of lye

For recipes using more than one type of oil, calculate the amount of lye needed for each oil, then add the lye amounts to get the total lye needed. Thankfully, lye calculators can do all the math for you, eliminating human error.

Calculating Lye and Water Discounts

Another reason to appreciate lye calculators is that they do the math for *superfatting* or *lye discounting* soaps. Both terms mean you are using less lye than normal. When you superfat your soap, you add extra oil but no extra lye; when you lye discount, you simply use less lye. Either way, you end up with a little bit of extra unsaponified oil in your finished soap, which creates a more luxurious, skin-pampering bar. But overdoing it reduces the lather and makes for a softer bar that doesn't last as long. A lye discount is typically less than 10 percent, meaning that less than 10 percent of the oil remains unsaponified in the final bar. The math for a 9 percent lye discount in a 100-ounce (2.8 kg) recipe with coconut oil looks like this:

SAP value (0.178) × amount of oil (100 ounces/ 2.8 kg) = 17.8 ounces (504 g) of lye × 0.91 (100–9) = 16.02 ounces (454 g) of lye

Unless you love doing math by hand, it's easier and more accurate to figure out your recipes using an online lye calculator.

Just as you can discount lye, you can discount water. In most recipes, water is the carrier for the lye. It also adds to the fluidity of the soap batter. If you discount the water in a batch, your soap will produce a harder bar more quickly because less water needs to evaporate from the end product, reducing curing time. Do not discount more than 40 percent; if you do, you may end up with undissolved lye crystals, and your batch could thicken extremely quickly.

Equipment Needed

For the most part, soap can be made with common kitchen equipment, so you don't need anything fancy to get started. You do need a scale and thermometer, however, and you should have a separate set of bowls, measuring cups, stirring implements, and the like that are used only for soaping.

Keep all soapmaking equipment separate from anything used for food preparation. That includes cleanup — wash soapmaking equipment by hand, not in the dishwasher. Here are the basic tools you'll need.

Protective wear. Keep your skin and eyes covered at all times while working with soap batter. You must have goggles (glasses do not offer enough protection), gloves (latex, nitrile, or rubber dishwashing gloves), long sleeves and pants, and closed-toe shoes. Cover your workspace with cardboard or several layers of newsprint.

Heat-resistant, nonreactive containers. Bowls and measuring cups made of tempered glass, stainless steel, or polypropylene plastic work best. (Aluminum reacts with lye to create toxic fumes and is not appropriate for soapmaking!) You need at least one large one (4 quarts/3.8 liters) for mixing batter.

Measuring bowls with spouts and handles are easier to use. Easy-pour containers with longer spouts are handy for creating complex patterns and color combinations.

Digital scale. Always measure ingredients by weight, not volume. Volume is not accurate enough to make soap with consistent quality. Digital scales are cheap, accurate, and easy to use; any that measures to a tenth of an ounce

(or about 2.8 grams) will work. Most models offer both metric and U.S. standard modes.

Thermometer. Temperature affects cold-process soap in many ways. Soap that is too hot can crack, volcano (bubble out of the mold), or develop "alien brain" (a weirdly textured top). If it's too cold, it can develop soda ash (see page 257). In order to have consistently successful batches of soap, a reliable thermometer is a must. This is especially true when testing the temperature of lye-water. A candy thermometer works fine, but I love using an infrared thermometer because it never touches the soap, so I don't need to clean it.

Stick or immersion blender. Mixing soap by hand can literally take hours. A stick blender makes quick work of emulsifying the lye and oils. A stainless steel shaft will last the longest, and a removable shaft helps with cleaning. Do not use your soapmaking stick blender for food preparation.

Whisk. It's useful to have whisks in several sizes for incorporating your additives, especially powders, which can clump. Whisks can also help achieve and maintain appropriate trace for the recipe.

Stainless steel spoons. These are handy for creating designs, mixing in additives, and more. Again, aluminum reacts with lye and *cannot* be used for soapmaking at any stage.

Rubber or silicone spatula. Use for scraping every last bit of soap out of your container into the mold.

Measuring cups and spoons. Most ingredients are added by weight, but these are used when adding colorants or other additives (such as sodium lactate, exfoliants, and salts).

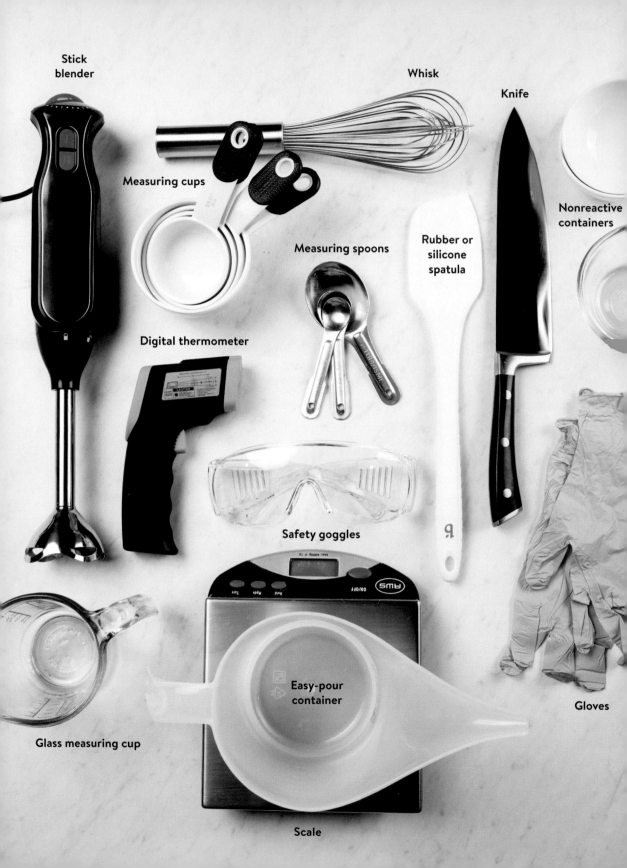

Stick blender

Whisk

Knife

Measuring cups

Nonreactive containers

Measuring spoons

Rubber or silicone spatula

Digital thermometer

Safety goggles

Gloves

Glass measuring cup

Easy-pour container

Scale

Small glass containers or bowls. These are helpful for weighing out smaller amounts of additives, like extracts, ahead of time.

Large knife or wire soap slicer. A sharp implement is needed for slicing finished loaves into bars. Multibar cutters are great for precise and even bars, but a good kitchen knife works fine.

Cutting board. Placing a cutting board under silicone molds before pouring in the batter helps stabilize the mold. The board also comes in handy for moving flexible silicone molds that need to be placed in the freezer to prevent overheating.

Soap molds. There are many options for soap molds. They are most commonly made of wood, plastic, or silicone. Do not use glass or aluminum molds to make soap. It is difficult to release the soap from a glass mold, and aluminum, as mentioned before, reacts with lye to make dangerous gases.

Choosing a Mold

Soaps can be molded into shapes as various as the colors and scents you can choose. A straightforward recipe can be made in anything from a lined shoebox to a cleaned-out yogurt tub. Most household containers that have some flexibility can be used for a soap mold.

Glass containers are not recommended for cold-process soap molds. For one thing, it is extremely hard to remove soap from them. Rigid molds should always be lined with freezer paper or a specially designed liner, otherwise you may never get the soap out! Never use metal containers for soaping, even if they are lined — again, lye reacts with many metals, especially aluminum, to create toxic fumes.

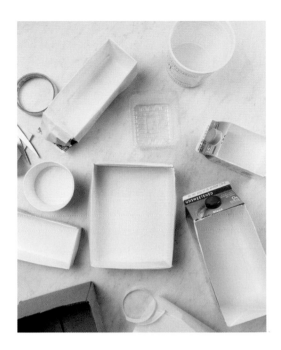

Recycled Molds

Pros: Create unique shapes, cost effective, eco-friendly

Cons: Inconsistent shapes, may require liners, typically good for just one use

Just about any container that held food or other nontoxic material can be turned into a soap mold with proper lining. If the container is plastic, the soap can be poured directly, without lining. Popular options include yogurt containers, pudding cups, and tofu containers. Cardboard milk containers are also a good option; the insides are normally lined with a nonstick coating. Recycling objects and boxes from home is a great way to save money on molds and create eco-friendly, unusual-looking bars.

On the downside, recycled molds may not be very sturdy and probably won't produce completely straight or uniform bars. Depending on the sturdiness of the container, it may be good for only one soaping recipe. And once used to make soap, the container cannot be reused for food storage. Containers used to make soap should be thrown away, not recycled.

Cardboard and other nonplastic containers need to be lined to ensure the soap does not stick or leak through. When soap is poured directly onto cardboard, it sticks and makes the cardboard soggy, resulting in a mess. But cardboard molds do work if you first line them with freezer paper, making sure that the shiny side faces the soap. Don't use wax paper; it isn't sturdy enough and will melt and stick to the soap.

Silicone Molds

Pros: Easy to unmold, easy to clean, don't require liners, last a long time, create professional-looking bars

Cons: Soap takes slightly longer to unmold, bubbles may form in bars if soap overheats

Silicone molds are easy to use and affordable. Sturdy yet flexible, silicone molds make unmolding both cold-process and melt-and-pour soap easy; the key is to break the airlock by gently pulling the sides of the mold away from the soap.

Soap takes longer to harden in silicone molds because air cannot contact the soap. In my opinion, the trade-off is worth it just for the time saved in not having to line the mold.

If you experience any resistance when removing cold-process soap, stop and give it a few more days in the mold. It's not worth tearing the sides or bottom of the project to get your soap out a little sooner.

In addition to easy unmolding, silicone molds are easy to care for. After removing the soap from the molds, hand-wash them with hot water and dish soap. (While silicone molds are sturdy, do not place them in the dishwasher.) Avoid any harsh scrubbing materials such as copper sponges; they may scratch the glossy inside finish. Allow to dry, and they are ready to use for the next project.

Using Sodium Lactate

Sodium lactate is a key additive when working with silicone molds. It is a liquid salt that helps the soap harden faster in the mold. This means that instead of waiting 3 or 4 days to unmold the project, the soap can often be unmolded the very next day. It also produces a harder bar of soap that lasts longer in the shower. The usage rate can vary, but in this book, 1 teaspoon (5 mL) of sodium lactate per pound (454 g) of soap is added directly to cooled lye-water.

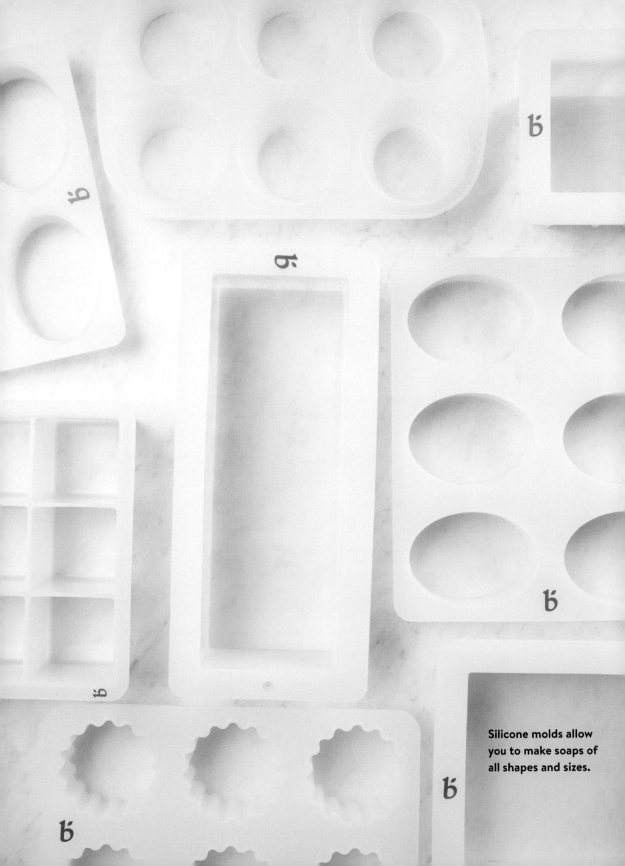

Silicone molds allow
you to make soaps of
all shapes and sizes.

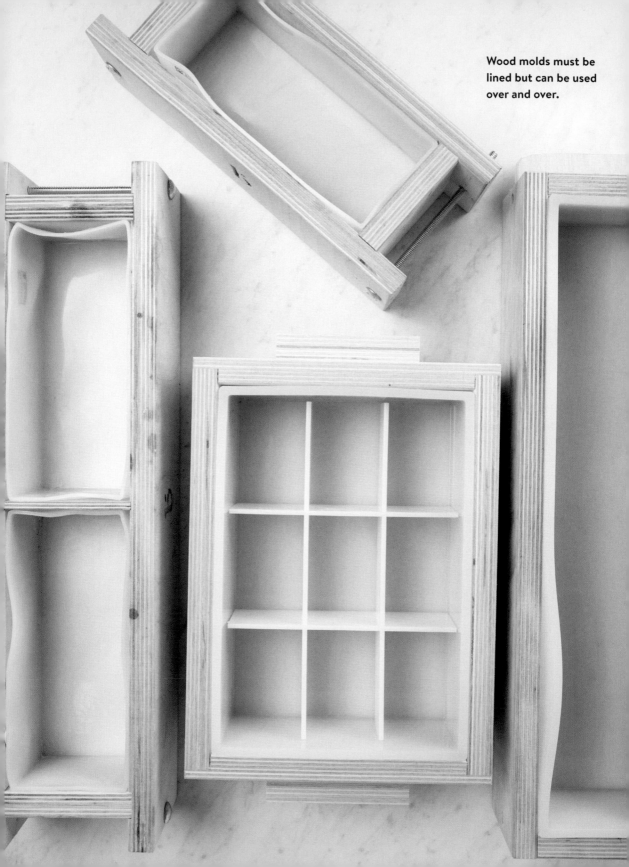

Wood molds must be lined but can be used over and over.

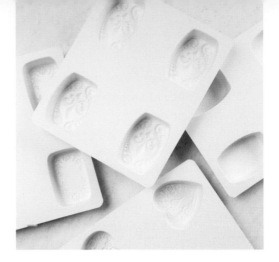

Wood Molds

Pros: Easy to insulate for gel phase, long lasting, produce large batches, professional-looking bars

Cons: Need to be lined, can soften over time, prone to overheating

Wood molds are sturdy, cost effective, and act as great insulators for cold-process soap. With proper storage and care, they can also last for years and years. Wooden molds come in all shapes and sizes. Common shapes are log (loaf), horizontal, slab, and divider molds.

Wood molds need to be lined with freezer paper to keep the soap from sticking. To make the unmolding process easier, many Bramble Berry wood molds are available with silicone liners, which saves a lot of time.

One of the best features of wood molds is that they insulate the soap well, making it easy to achieve a complete gel phase through-out the soap. It's important to keep this in mind when insulating wood molds; because they insulate naturally, placing the mold on a heating pad to achieve gel phase may not be necessary. (On the other hand, to avoid gel phase completely, place the mold and soap in the refrigerator or other cool place.)

Plastic Molds

Pros: Wide variety of shapes and designs, cost effective, great for small batches, create professional-looking bars

Cons: Can be difficult and time consuming to unmold, prone to soda ash, not as suitable for making large batches

While best suited for melt-and-pour soap making, plastic molds can also be used for cold-process soap. They come in a wide variety of shapes and sizes: if it can be imagined, there is probably a plastic mold for it. The majority of plastic molds are for individual soaps, usually 4 to 6 ounces (113–170 mL). The smaller size means that the molds do not insulate the soap as well as large slab or loaf molds. Do not place plastic molds on a heating pad because they might melt or warp.

Instead of using gel phase to help prevent soda ash, you can spritz the soap with 99% rubbing (isopropyl) alcohol several times over a time span of 90 minutes. This creates a protective barrier on top of the soap. Another option is to decrease the superfat level to 3 percent or water discount at 10 percent.

Removing cold-process soap from plastic molds can be a bit tricky and can require up to a week. If you must use a plastic mold, incorporate a large amount of hard oils (such as palm oil, coconut oil, or cocoa butter) in the recipe to help the soap harden. Adding sodium lactate also helps, and some soapers lubricate their molds with a unsaponifiable liquid such as cyclomethicone (a liquid silicone and common cosmetic additive) or mineral oil. Additionally, using a trace that is too thick can make it difficult to achieve good details with intricate molds.

Safety

Sodium hydroxide (lye) is an inorganic compound commonly found in drain cleaners. It is highly caustic, and it can burn your skin or blind you. Because lye has the potential to be extremely dangerous, it's important to take every safety precaution when making cold-process soap.

Sodium hydroxide is available in various forms, commonly flakes, pellets, or powder. To make cold-process soap, lye is introduced to a liquid, usually distilled water. The liquid dissolves the lye and creates a solution. Mixing water and lye also creates an exothermic reaction, with a dramatic increase in temperature. Adding lye to room-temperature water can raise the water's temperature up to 200°F (93°C). The mixture also creates toxic fumes that should not be inhaled.

Precautions for Soaping Safely

Wear proper safety gear. When working with lye, wearing protective safety gear is not an option — it's a must. This includes eye goggles, gloves, long sleeves, long pants, and closed-toe shoes. Covering your skin helps protect it from spills or splashes of lye solution. Some soapers also like to wear surgical masks or full-face masks. Sodium hydroxide has a high pH and can burn skin, ruin wood surfaces, and damage eyes. *The most important safety equipment is your goggles — eyeglasses are not enough.*

It's important to wear your safety gear during the entire soapmaking process. Lye

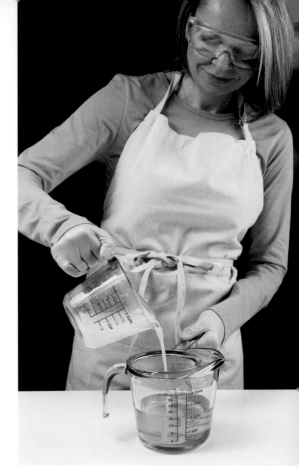

Never make soap without taking all the necessary safety precautions. Wearing an apron offers extra protection.

solution can irritate the skin and eyes even when mixed with soaping oils. Raw soap batter is not as dangerous as pure lye-water, but it can still irritate the skin; wearing safety gear while soaping helps avoid any contact with it. You can get soap batter on your skin and not notice until several minutes later, when your skin begins to tingle and burn.

Quickly wash away any soap batter on the skin with water and (ironically) a gentle soap. Once saponification is complete, all lye molecules have been transformed into soap, and the batter will no longer harm the skin.

Mix lye in an appropriate place. The area in which you mix the lye solution should have excellent ventilation to help you avoid breathing in fumes. When weather allows, many soapers like to mix their lye solution outside. Indoors, I like to open a few windows and/or turn on a fan. Some soapers prefer to soap with a ventilator or air filter on to help blow away any fumes that are created during the mixing process. It's also important to eliminate any other distractions or potential hazards; kids and pets should be kept out of the area, and the space should be cleared of all tripping hazards and other dangers.

Always add lye to water, never water to lye! When mixing water and lye, the first step is to measure the correct amounts into two separate containers. Once you have the correct amounts for your recipe measured out, the lye should be *slowly* added to the water. NEVER add water to lye! Doing so can cause the lye to erupt out of the container — and maybe into your face.

Use an appropriate mixing container. It's important to mix lye solution in a durable container made of sturdy, heat-resistant plastic or glass. Do not mix the lye solution in a metal container, for two reasons. First, the lye solution gets incredibly hot. Second, as I've mentioned,

First Aid

If you get lye on your skin: Immediately remove any contaminated clothing and flush skin with water for at least 15 minutes. Seek medical attention. If it comes in contact with eyes, flush immediately with water for at least 15 minutes and get medical attention. If fumes are inhaled, move to fresh air.

Many soapers keep vinegar on hand in the belief it neutralizes lye burns. There is controversy in the soapmaking community about washing lye burns with vinegar rather than water. According to the sodium hydroxide MSDS (Material Safety Data Sheet), wash with plain water. Adding vinegar (a weak acid) to lye (a strong base) creates a chemical reaction that releases more heat, so putting vinegar on a lye burn just plain hurts. I'd stick with water.

Although vinegar should not be used to treat lye burns on skin, it *can* be used as a precaution during the cleanup process. A quick wipe of your workspace with a vinegar-soaked rag will neutralize any lye dust that may have gotten on the surface.

If you accidentally swallow lye or lye-water, do not induce vomiting. Lye is extremely corrosive and will burn the mouth, tongue, throat, esophagus, and lungs on the way down — and on the way back up if vomiting is induced. If you or someone in your household swallows lye, do not treat or manage it. Call the national toll-free Poison Help line (1-800-222-1222) and immediately get to a hospital. If the individual can swallow and is not having convulsions, have him or her drink water or milk while waiting for the ambulance or on the way to the hospital.

lye reacts hazardously with some metals. Sodium hydroxide and aluminum produce explosive hydrogen gas. Lye also reacts with tin, so avoid metal containers entirely.

If you're using a glass container, make sure it's extremely sturdy. I have used Pyrex containers successfully for years, but some soapers have had problems with them breaking. Choose a container that is large enough to catch any splashes as you stir with a stainless steel or silicone spoon. If you are at all nervous about this step, mix the lye and water over a sink in case there are any spills.

Store Lye Appropriately

While waiting for the lye solution to cool to suitable soaping temperatures, make sure your container is clearly labeled "LYE" to ensure nobody touches or tampers with the solution. It's also important to move it somewhere kids or pets will not touch or drink the solution. The jar of dry lye flakes, pellets, or powder should always be kept out of reach of children and should be properly labeled "POISON" and/or "DO NOT TOUCH" to ensure people do not tamper with it.

Because of lye's propensity to draw moisture from the air, airtight, chemical-resistant plastic containers work best. Lye is highly corrosive and can eat away at glass over time. Old lye sometimes acts as though it is not working. This is often because the lye has taken on so much moisture that when it is weighed out, it is significantly heavier with water weight than lye weight.

Cleanup Procedures

After you're done soaping, it's time to wash your dishes. Because raw soap can still irritate skin, leave your gloves on while washing any soaping dishes. Wipe out any excess soap with a paper towel, then wash your dishes in the sink with hot water and grease-cutting soap, like Dawn.

If you want to avoid washing oils down the sink, you may prefer the garbage bag cleanup method: scrape all of the soapy, greasy, semisolid mixture into a garbage bag, seal it tightly, and throw the entire thing away. If your septic system is delicate, this is a better choice for cleanup.

Basic
Cold-Process Recipe

It is key to have a strong understanding of soapmaking and how soap should look and act before you start making milk soap. Milk complicates soapmaking, so this beginner recipe uses water instead. If you've never made soap before, try making a few batches of this soap first so you know what to expect when you start experimenting with the addition of milk.

Before you start, please read all the safety instructions and set up your workspace in a well-ventilated area. Always suit up with gloves, goggles, long sleeves, long pants, and closed-toe shoes.

This basic recipe uses a 4-inch (10 cm) silicone loaf mold and produces four hard bars that lather well.

Oil Amounts
3.6 ounces/102 g
  palm oil (30%)
3.6 ounces/102 g
  coconut oil (30%)
3.6 ounces/102 g
  olive oil (30%)
1.2 ounces/34 g
  sweet almond oil (10%)

Lye-Water
3.9 ounces/111 g
  distilled water
1.7 ounces/48 g
  lye (5% superfat)
1 teaspoon/5 mL
  sodium lactate

Fragrance Oil
0.8 ounce/23 g Energy

Colorant
1 teaspoon/5 mL yellow
  oxide dispersed into
  1 tablespoon/15 mL
  sweet almond oil (See
  Dispersing Additives in
  Oil, page 46)

For more information on the soapmaking process,
see the glossary (page 257) and FAQ section (page 258).

1. Measure the lye-water

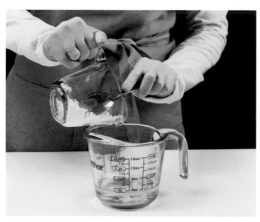

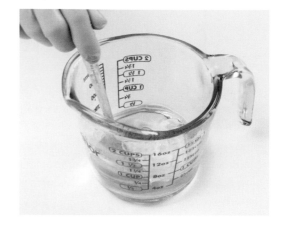

Weigh the distilled water and the lye into separate heatproof containers. Add the lye *slowly* to the water. (Never add water to lye or it may erupt like a volcano!)

Using a stainless steel spoon, stir by hand to dissolve the lye; be careful not to splash. Stir at arm's length to avoid breathing the fumes. Stir until the water turns clear.

2. Measure the oils

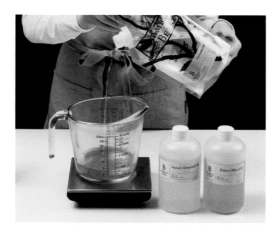

Palm and coconut oil are both generally solid at room temperature and need to be melted before being measured. Palm oil separates as it cools, so it must also be mixed before measuring to ensure consistency. Melt both oils in their original containers on low heat in the microwave. Measure the olive oil and the sweet almond oil into a heatproof bowl large enough to hold the entire batch of soap batter. Mix the palm oil thoroughly and measure it into the bowl. Measure the coconut oil into the bowl, stir the oils together, and set the mixture aside.

3. Mix the soap

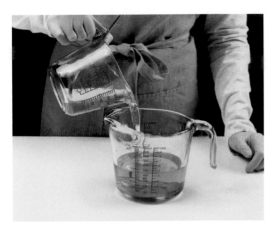

Let both the oil mixture and lye-water mixture cool to between 120 and 130°F (49–54°C). You can place them into ice baths to cool more quickly. If the oils become too cool, you can warm them on low in the microwave. Never microwave lye-water.

Add the sodium lactate to the lye-water now and stir well. (This additive isn't required, but I recommend it for most recipes, as it allows for quicker and easier unmolding.)

Pour the lye-water carefully and slowly into your melted oils.

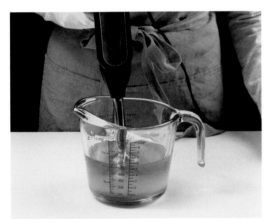

Insert the stick blender into the batter, tilting it or tapping it against the bottom of the bowl so that any trapped air can escape. With the blades fully immersed, turn the blender on low. *Never turn on the stick blender until the blades are fully immersed.* Move the blender around the bowl slowly, taking care to keep the blades of the stick blender submerged.

TECHNIQUE TIP

Pouring the lye-water over the back of a spatula or the shaft of the stick blender avoids creating bubbles and reduces the risk of splashing.

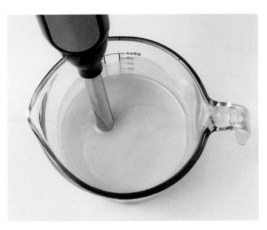

You will see the emulsification process start as the mixture goes from an oil-and-water suspension to a thicker, opaque batter that is a light ivory/yellow color.

4. Achieving trace

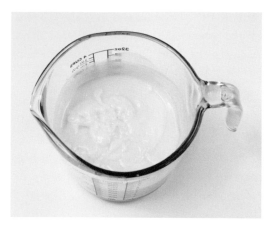

At this point, start looking for "trace." This is when you can trace a design on the surface of the mixture by drizzling batter onto it from the head of your switched-off stick blender; the trace of your drizzle should remain on the surface as a faint outline for a few seconds. This is the visual sign that the soap has emulsified to the point where you can add your fragrance, colorants, herbs, and other additives.

5. Add fragrance and colorant

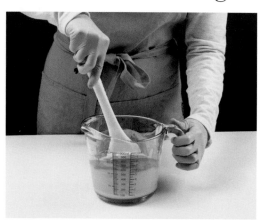

Add the fragrance oil and 1 teaspoon (5 mL) of the premixed yellow oxide, and stir in by hand with a spatula or whisk. (Using a stick blender now will overly thicken the trace.)

6. Pour into the mold

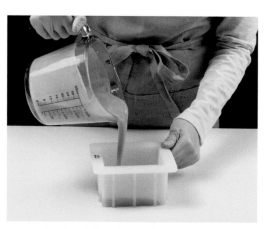

After your additives have been thoroughly mixed in, pour the soap batter into the mold. (This recipe's silicone mold needs no prepping or lining.)

7. Spray the soap

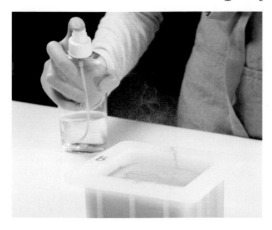

Spray the top of the soap thoroughly with 99% isopropyl alcohol several times over the next 90 minutes. (This step isn't required, but it prevents the buildup of harmless but unsightly soda ash on the soap as it cures.)

Cover the mold and insulate it with a towel for 12 to 24 hours to encourage gel phase (see page 257). Unwrap the mold and let it sit for an additional 2 to 4 days before releasing it from the mold. The longer the soap sits, the harder it becomes and the easier it will be to unmold.

8. Unmold and cut

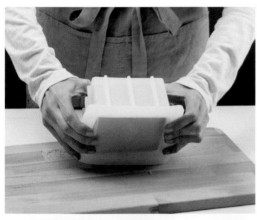

The loaf of finished soap should be the consistency of refrigerated butter. If it is too soft, or if it isn't releasing easily from the mold, let it sit for an additional 1 or 2 days and check it again. After you unmold it, cut the soap into bars with a sharp, nonserrated knife or a soap cutter.

Lay the bars on a wire cooling rack that allows for air circulation. Make sure they aren't touching. Let the sliced bars cure in a well-ventilated area out of direct sunlight for 4 to 6 weeks before using, turning them every few days to ensure they cure evenly.

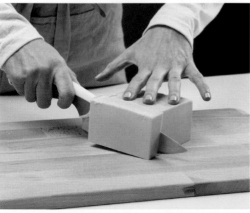

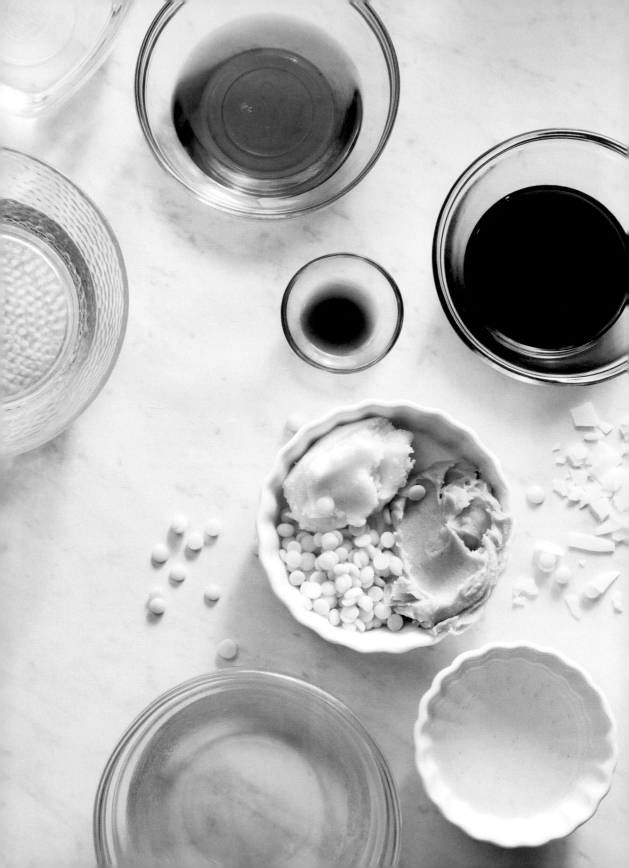

CHAPTER THREE

Properties of Different Oils

In addition to providing the fat that saponifies and becomes soap, oils add important properties. Each oil brings different characteristics to the final bar of soap. For example, if you want your soap to be conditioning, you might choose avocado oil or shea butter. If you'd like lots of lather, try using coconut and palm oil, or adding some castor oil.

Here are brief descriptions of the oils used in this book; there are many others. Note that some oils, called "hard oils," are solid at room temperature or below; these must be melted before being combined with lye. Store oils properly. Oils with a short shelf life are more prone to going rancid, which can discolor finished soaps. It's fun to experiment with different oils to find the ones that you like best.

Apricot kernel oil (SAP VALUE: 0.135)

Apricot kernel oil is high in fatty acids and vitamins A, C, and E. Being high in unsaturated fat, it has amazing conditioning and moisturizing properties but does not help with cleansing or bar hardness. Apricot kernel oil is typically used at 15 percent or below.

Argan oil (SAP VALUE: 0.135)

Argan oil contains vitamins A and E. It also contains squalene, a natural emollient and antioxidant. Argan oil is commonly used to boost moisture in soap and is usually used at 10 percent or below.

Avocado butter (SAP VALUE: 0.133)

Avocado butter is hydrogenated and ranges in color from ivory to soft green. It has a mild odor. It feels great on the skin and adds a gentle nourishing touch to soap. Avocado butter is typically used at 15 percent or less.

Avocado oil (SAP VALUE: 0.133)

Avocado oil varies in color from green to yellow, but this has little effect on the color of the final product. Avocado oil adds conditioning and moisturizing properties and is usually used at 20 percent or below.

Babassu oil (SAP VALUE: 0.179)

Babassu oil, which comes from a Brazilian palm tree, is a great replacement for either coconut or palm oil. It contributes the same firming and moisturizing properties and acts similarly by enhancing lather and adding hardness. Babassu does have a lighter feeling on the skin, and it absorbs quickly. It can also accelerate trace. It is most often used at 30 percent or below.

Borage oil (SAP VALUE: 0.133)

This oil is great for sensitive or mature skin. It is a very rich source of essential fatty acids, including gamma-linolenic acid, which helps nourish and hydrate the skin. Borage oil has a shorter shelf life than many others and is expensive. Because of this, it is used at 3 percent or less in most soap recipes.

Canola oil (SAP VALUE: 0.133)

Canola oil is an economical, neutral soaping oil that is fantastic for recipes that need a lot of working time or when a neutral color is desired. High-oleic canola oil is the best choice, as it will not go rancid as quickly as regular canola oil. Canola oil is best used with hard oils such as coconut and palm oil. It can be used up to 40 percent.

Considering Nut Allergies

When making soap for other people, it's important to be aware of nut allergies. Individuals with severe allergies can have serious reactions to nut-based oils. When labeling soap for sale, make sure to list every ingredient used in the soap — including carrier oils, oils used to disperse colorants, and additives, such as ground nut shells used for exfoliation — to keep customers with allergies safe.

Castor oil (SAP VALUE: 0.128)

This thick, sticky oil has a distinctive odor, but don't worry, it disappears in the final bars. Its light yellow color generally won't affect the color of the final product. Castor oil creates large, luxurious bubbles but is used at 8 percent or below to avoid tackiness in the final bar.

Chia seed oil (SAP VALUE: 0.160)

Chia seed oil is very high in omega-3 fatty acid, making it a popular additive for hair, skin, and nail products. It contains over 57 percent alpha-linolenic fatty acids, which add soothing and conditioning properties. It's marketed for its antioxidant benefits and vitamins A, B_1, B_2, B_3, niacin, iron, and zinc. Chia seed oil has a soothing, nutty aroma that won't transfer to the final soap. It is most often used at 15 percent or below.

Cocoa butter (SAP VALUE: 0.137)

Cocoa butter has a distinctively nutty, chocolaty aroma that may come through in the finished soap. Despite its name, it has a hard and crumbly consistency and must be melted before being mixed with lye-water. Cocoa butter comes in two forms, deodorized and natural. The deodorized version, often called "Maria grade," is usually whiter than natural cocoa butter and does not smell like chocolate. Cocoa butter contributes to bar hardness. If it's used over 15 percent, the soap may become difficult to cut and be prone to cracking.

Coconut oil (SAP VALUE: 0.118)

Coconut oil is expeller-pressed from the meat of coconuts, then bleached and deodorized. Coconut oil extracted with solvents is less desirable. Coconut oil creates lather with large bubbles and helps to cut down on oils and grease. Its long shelf life and high stability make it a staple in soapmaking.

Coconut oil is solid at room temperature and must be melted before being measured for a recipe. Different formulations have different melt points: 76°F (24°C), 96°F (35.5°C), 101°F (38°C), and 110°F (43°C). They all work for soap, but the 76°F (24°C) version is the most commonly used for soap. It has a high cleansing ability, so some find it harsh on the skin if used above 25 percent.

Coffee butter (SAP VALUE: 0.132)

Coffee butter, a blend of coffee seed oil and hydrogenated vegetable oils, is a soft, luxurious butter that smells like a slightly burned cup of coffee. Pale brown in color, it can impart a lovely natural tan color to soap, as well as a subtle roasted-coffee scent. Coffee butter contains between 0.5 and 1 percent caffeine, which probably won't perk you up much. It has a shelf life of about one year. It does not contribute much to the lather or hardness of the bar but is very moisturizing. It is typically used at 10 percent or less.

Hazelnut oil (SAP VALUE: 0.137)

Hazelnut oil is nongreasy and gentle on the skin. It's a great moisturizer and adds conditioning and nourishing properties to soap. It works well combined with other oils. It has a short shelf life, so if you superfat with it, it may go rancid in soap that isn't used within a few months.

Hempseed oil (SAP VALUE: 0.135)

Hempseed (or hemp) oil does not contain tetrahydrocannabinol (THC), the psychoactive constituent found in the flowers. Depending on the degree of refining, its color varies from light yellow to dark green. Unrefined (green) hempseed oil can affect the final color of the bars depending on how much is used and how the batch is colored. It is used in skin-care products because of its high proportion of essential fatty acids. In soap, it provides a nourishing yet small lather. Unrefined hemp-seed oil has a short shelf life of 3 to 6 months. Refined hempseed oil keeps for 12 months. It is mostly used at 20 percent or less.

Jojoba oil (SAP VALUE: 0.069)

This oil is a liquid wax with a wonderful absorption rate and moisturizing abilities. Jojoba oil has a very long shelf life, as its fatty acids help resist oxidation and rancidity. It is typically used at under 8 percent.

Kokum butter (SAP VALUE: 0.135)

Kokum butter is a firm, highly emollient butter with a light, nongreasy texture. It melts just above body temperature, and skin and hair absorb it readily, restoring softness and elasticity. It is one of the most stable vegetable butters against oxidation. Most kokum butters are expeller-pressed and then refined, bleached, and deodorized. It's typically used at 15 percent or less.

Kukui nut oil (SAP VALUE: 0.135)

The kukui (koo-koo-ee) nut is also known as the candlenut (the oil is also used in making candles). The oil is pricey, but it penetrates skin beautifully, leaving it feeling silky and smooth; it's a luxurious addition to soap. It's mostly used at 6 percent or less.

Macadamia nut oil

(SAP VALUE: 0.194)

Macadamia nut oil is often used in soap and cosmetics to replace mink oil, which many people prefer to avoid. Macadamia nut oil provides conditioning and moisturizing qual-ities. It is stable in soapmaking, although it does not produce copious bubbles. Because it does not contribute much to bar hardness or lather, it is used at 10 percent or less in most recipes.

Mango butter (SAP VALUE: 0.184)

Mango butter is refined, bleached, and deodorized until it is ivory in color, with a creamy texture. In soap, it adds conditioning and nourishing properties. It is typically used at 15 percent or less.

Matcha green tea butter

(SAP VALUE: 0.130)

Matcha is a traditional Japanese tea known for its abundant antioxidants. This butter is a mixture of sweet almond oil and hydrogenated vegetable oil with *Camellia sinensis* (tea) leaf powder added to it. It is very skin-loving and a great addition to cold-process soap when used at 10 percent or below.

Meadowfoam oil (SAP VALUE: 0.120)

Meadowfoam oil is unusual in having almost 100 percent long-chain fatty acids, which makes it extremely emollient and moisturiz-ing. Meadowfoam lasts up to three years in a refrigerator. Because it does not add to bar hardness or lather, it is used at 20 percent or less. Using more produces a slightly softer bar with smaller bubbles.

Neem oil (SAP VALUE: 0.137)

Neem has a very distinctive scent that can be described as musky or garlicky. It is also normally a yellowish brown color. In spite of the odor and color, this oil has been used for centuries because of its perceived moisturizing abilities and high amount of antioxidants. Depending on how much is used, this oil may add a nutty, earthy smell to the final soap. With its long shelf life, it can be used in many soap projects. It is typically used at under 6 percent.

Olive oil (SAP VALUE: 0.134)

Olive oil is available in a variety of grades. While extra-virgin olive oil is not necessary for soap recipes, it is important to use a pure grade. Some methods of extraction, such as the last pressing, use chemical solvents that may end up in the final product; they can accelerate trace.

Extra-virgin olive oil (a.k.a. "pure" olive oil) allows a long working time and is a staple for designs with complicated swirls, lots of different colors, or accelerating essential oils, such as cinnamon. If a recipe calls for olive oil, do not substitute with olive pomace oil, which is made by extracting the last bits of oil from the paste left over after pressing extra-virgin olive oil. It contains high percentages of unsaponifiables and is known to speed up trace. This oil is used when a recipe needs to set up slightly sooner, such as in some of the layering projects or recipes that have a textured top. Extra-virgin olive oil can be substituted in these recipes, but be aware that trace will be delayed.

All types of olive oil produce exceptionally mild soap with small bubbles, suitable for sensitive skin and babies. Unlike most other oils, it can be used up to 100 percent in soap recipes; soap made from 100 percent olive oil is called castile soap. When fresh, the lather is slick.

Olive oil soap needs a longer time to cure (up to 8 weeks) but the bars age beautifully; the lather and hardness improve over time. Note: "Light" olive oil doesn't work in soap at all.

Palm kernel oil (SAP VALUE: 0.178)

Palm kernel oil (PKO) is obtained from the kernel (the edible seed) of the oil palm fruit. PKO comes as flakes and is solid at room temperature. It contains highly saturated fats that contribute to bar hardness and lather stability. When used at amounts higher than 15 percent in soap, it will accelerate trace, and the soap can become brittle and waxy.

Palm oil (SAP VALUE: 0.144)

Palm oil comes from the pulp of the fruit from palm trees. In soap, palm oil helps to stabilize lather, adds hardness, and acts as a secondary lathering agent. Used in conjunction with coconut oil, it creates large bubbles that last. Palm

Vitamin E Oil

Though technically an oil, vitamin E oil does not saponify and is used as an additive after the batter is mixed. An excellent antioxidant, this thick oil helps slow the oxidizing process that can cause soap to go rancid. It is easy to use in recipes and helps extend the shelf life of soap.

Palm oil, *continued*

oil is solid at room temperature and must be fully melted and mixed before being measured for a recipe. Because of its hardening ability, keep it to 25 percent or less of your recipe.

For soapmaking, choose RBD (refined, bleached, and deodorized) palm oil. Palm oil is becoming increasingly controversial because of its environmental impact, so look for palm oil that is certified sustainable by the Roundtable on Sustainable Palm Oil.

Pumpkin seed oil (SAP VALUE: 0.138)

This cold-pressed oil has a warm aroma and striking dark color that is unlikely to affect the color of the final bars. It contains vitamins A and E, as well as linoleic (omega-6) fatty acids, all skin-loving ingredients. This lightweight oil adds conditioning properties to soap without weighing down the lather. It is most often used at 10 percent or less.

Rice bran oil (SAP VALUE: 0.129)

Rice bran oil is derived from the outer layers of rice grains, which are packed with antioxidants, essential fatty acids, and vitamin E.

It produces a small, mild lather, similar to olive oil lather, and can be used in place of olive oil to save money. Though it can be used in cold-process recipes up to 100 percent, it is used at 50 percent or below in most.

Safflower oil (SAP VALUE: 0.135)

Safflower oil is an inexpensive oil that is moisturizing in soap and creates a mild, low lather. It can be used interchangeably with sunflower or canola oil (after running through a lye calculator). Standard safflower oil has a fairly short shelf life of one year, so look for the high-oleic version, which lasts longer. It can be used up to 20 percent in recipes.

Shea butter (SAP VALUE: 0.128)

Unrefined shea butter is gray and smells smoky, but when fully refined it turns creamy and white. Shea butter has great moisturizing abilities, and because it is a well-known ingredient, it provides ample label appeal. It is not a good lathering agent on its own and will speed up trace. It is typically used at 10 percent or below.

━━━ Using Animal Fat Instead of Oil ━━━

Animal fats have been used in place of vegetable oils for hundreds of years in soapmaking to produce hard, white bars of soap with mild, creamy lather. Tallow and lard, from beef and pork respectively, are the most commonly used, although soapers have been known to use more exotic fats, such as bear or beaver.

Different animal fats have slightly different SAP values, though they generally fall within a range of 0.134 to 0.141. Tallow has a SAP value of 0.138 to 0.141; lard's is 0.139 to 0.141. There are a few outliers, such as lanolin (0.075) and mink oil (0.160). Always check the exact SAP value for any fat or use a lye calculator; small differences in SAP value can have a big effect on the amount of lye needed to neutralize your soap.

Shea oil (SAP VALUE: 0.129)

Shea oil is fractionated (separated) shea butter. It has all the same benefits but is easier to work with, as you don't have to melt it before measuring. It is high in oleic acid, which some consider to be anti-inflammatory, as well as high in linoleic acid, which is key to skin repair. Because shea oil is lower in stearic acid than shea butter, it does not contribute to bar hardness. Additionally, it is high in unsaponifiables, so it is mostly used at 8 percent or less.

Sunflower oil (SAP VALUE: 0.134)

Sunflower oil is full of essential fatty acids and vitamin E, which condition and moisturize skin. It has a short shelf life, so either keep it in the refrigerator or look for high-oleic versions, which tend to be more stable. When combined with olive and palm oil, it produces a rich, creamy lather. Use sunflower oil at less than 20 percent or it will result in a soft soap.

Sweet almond oil (SAP VALUE: 0.136)

Sweet almond oil has many vitamins, including A, B_6, and E. It contributes to conditioning and moisturizing skin but will make softer bars. It has a shelf life of 9 to 12 months and is typically used at 25 percent or less.

Tamanu oil (SAP VALUE: 0.144)

The thick green oil of the tropical tamanu tree has been used for centuries for medicinal purposes and skin care. It takes 220 pounds (100 kg) of tamanu fruit, the annual production of one adult tree, to make just 11 pounds (5 kg) of cold-pressed tamanu oil. Use it in soap up to 5 percent.

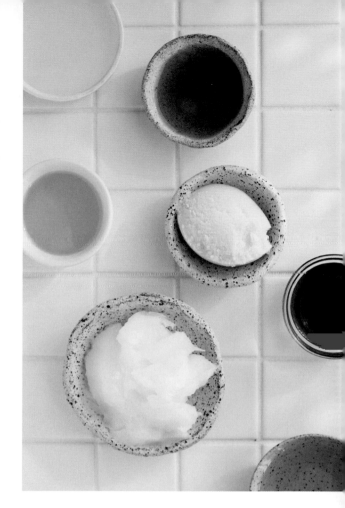

Wheat germ oil (SAP VALUE: 0.133)

Wheat germ oil contains many nutrients, including vitamins A, B, D, and E. It has a light and powdery feeling on the skin, which makes it an excellent component of cold-process face soap. This cold-pressed oil has a dark yellow color and a nutty, oaty scent. The color may or may not affect the final result, depending on how much is used and what the color scheme is. When used at 10 percent or less and with a strong fragrance, the odor isn't as noticeable.

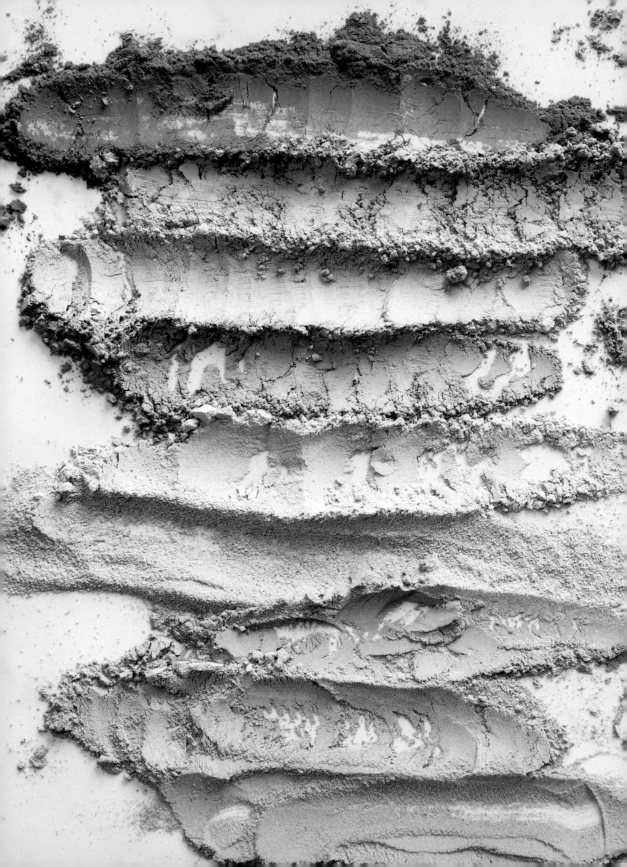

CHAPTER FOUR

Adding
Color & Scent

Soapmaking is a science first, but it becomes an art when we choose a design and add colors, fragrances, essential oils, and exfoliants or other ingredients to create something beyond a plain white bath bar. From a range of creamy natural tones to a dazzling array of bright colors, you can make soap in just about any color and pattern you can imagine. Plus you can add a strong, long-lasting scent to your soap with pure essential oils or specially formulated fragrance oils.

Adding Color

Coloring soap is a fantastic way to show your personality, develop a distinctive style, and, if you're planning to sell your soap, attract people to your product. After all, a beautifully colored, attractively designed soap is sure to catch the eye of most passersby. Color can also enhance the scent of your soap. People are more likely to say, "Mm, this smells like strawberry!" about a bar of gorgeous pink soap than a plain white one.

The Food and Drug Administration (FDA), which is responsible for regulating all color additives, defines color additives as "any dye, pigment or substances which when added or applied to a food, drug or cosmetic, or to the human body, is capable (alone or through reactions with other substances) of imparting color." There are a variety of options for coloring soap. Manufactured colorants include food, drug, and cosmetic (FD&C) colors and synthetic micas (shiny silicate minerals). Natural colorants include oxides and pigments, clays, herbs, and some micas.

Using Oxides (Pigments)

Oxides, also referred to as pigments, are a class of colorants that have been used for centuries to color soap. In the past, most were derived from natural sources, but today most pigments are made in laboratories; even pigments that are mined from the earth must be purified before they can be used in soapmaking. Oxides are used in many applications, from paint to car finishes to cosmetics. They are generally stable and can withstand high heat, high levels of pH, and exposure to light.

While oxides are technically all natural, since they come from the ground, they are not necessarily eco-friendly. They are often contaminated with heavy metals and require multiple purification steps, and there is considerable environmental impact in mining them. But we are finding better ways. Ultramarine blue, for example, was originally made from lapis lazuli, an expensive, semiprecious stone. The modern equivalent is made from aluminum silicate with sulfur. It's still entirely natural and produces a beautiful, pure blue.

Oxides are wonderful to work with in cold-process soap because they are typically stable in color, so what you see in the beginning is what you get at the end. Pigment and oxide clumps in soap will streak and can stain washcloths and skin, so it's important to mix them properly. To add them to soap, premix each teaspoon (5 mL) of pigment with 1 tablespoon (15 mL) of oil to work out clumps and ensure a smooth mixture.

Note: The pigments used in these recipes are from Bramble Berry. Other brands use different names for their colors. They will work fine but may produce a different color than shown.

Using Micas

Mica is a mineral that can be mined from the earth or synthesized in a factory. Crushed into powder, it reflects light like a diamond, adding sparkle and shine to cosmetic products. Micas give cold-process soap sheen and luminescence when wet.

In its natural state, mica is dull white or gray. When the particles are coated with a

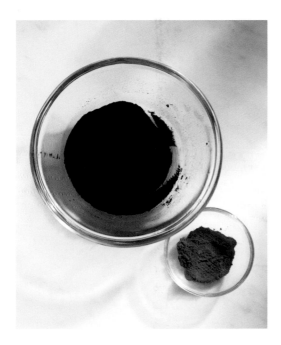

worth of shade and hue. FD&C colorants are most commonly derived from petroleum, though they can also be created from coal tar. They can be classified as dyes (which dissolve in water) or lakes (which do not).

In soap, FD&C colorants typically produce bright, vibrant colors. Because of the pH in the raw soap mixture, however, some FD&C colorants morph and produce unexpected results. For example, Blue No. 1 morphs from beautiful blue to purple when you mix it into the batter. Other colors may go from red to brown or from green to no color at all.

When experimenting with FD&C colorants in your soap, always check to see what color they will turn in the soap (your supplier should be able to tell you that) or do a small test batch to make sure the final outcome is what you were expecting. FD&C colorants for soaps, cosmetics, and toiletries are sold under the brand name Labcolors.

colorant, that color takes on mica's reflective sparkle. The finer the mica particles are, the more sparkle the color has. Mica can be considered all natural or synthetic depending on what the particles are coated with.

Mica coated with a pigment is considered a natural product. It is also colorfast, and the hue will not morph in soap. A mica coated with an FD&C colorant is not considered a natural product, and it may or may not be colorfast. It may morph and bleed in soap. Micas can be added directly at thin trace or premixed with oil to remove clumps.

Using FD&C Colorants

Synthetic FD&C colorants are more commonly known as food coloring. They are commercially manufactured, which makes them generally less expensive than all-natural alternatives. Additionally, their shelf life is often indefinite, and they can produce colors in a rainbow's

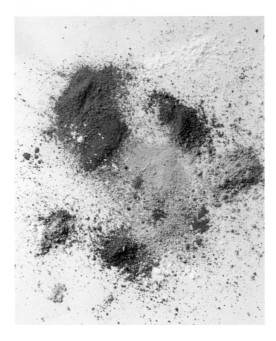

DIFFERENT SHADES OF MILK

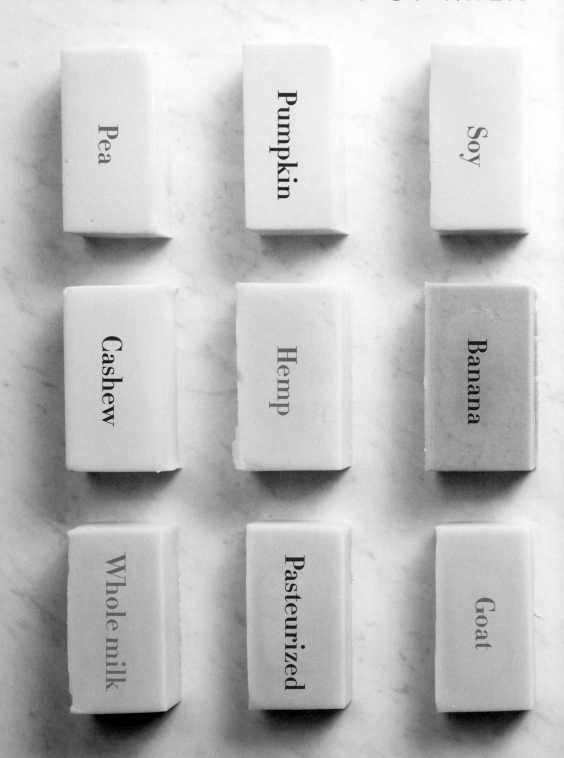

Pea

Pumpkin

Soy

Cashew

Hemp

Banana

Whole milk

Pasteurized

Goat

Milk soap can present a coloration challenge. Without added colorant, some milks will turn bright yellow, others light tan, and still others more of a gray. Overcoloring this natural palette is possible by choosing a base color that complements the natural color of the soap and incorporating both colors into an interesting design.

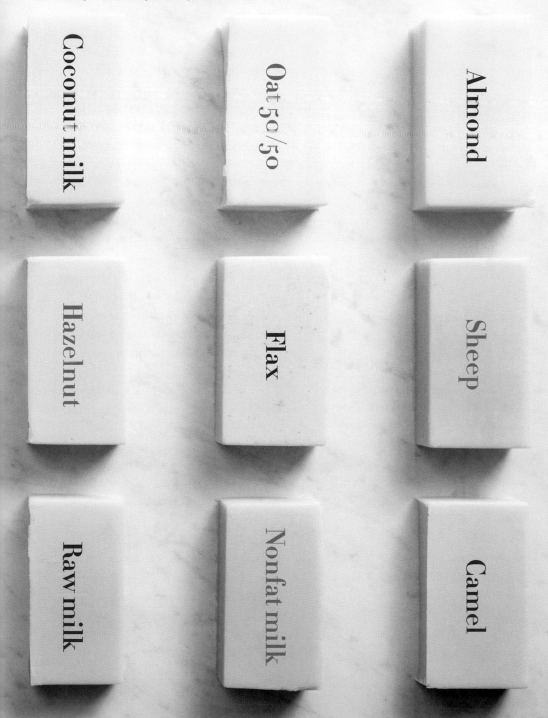

Coconut milk

Oat 50/50

Almond

Hazelnut

Flax

Sheep

Raw milk

Nonfat milk

Camel

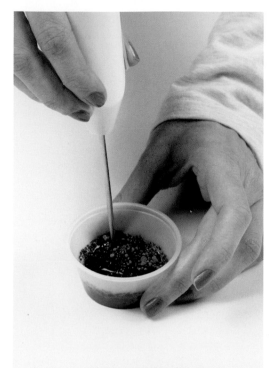

Dispersing Additives in Oil

Most colorants and other additives must be mixed with a small amount of oil before being combined with the soap batter. This ensures that they are evenly distributed, with no clumps. The rate is typically 1 teaspoon (5 mL) of powder dispersed in 1 tablespoon (15 mL) of oil, then measured out as called for in the recipe. A mini blender or milk frother does a great job, but you can also mix them by hand using a small whisk.

Using Other Additives for Color

Various herbs, herbal infusions, botanicals, clays, and powders can give soap surprisingly vibrant hues.

Herbs used in soap must be cosmetic grade or food grade. (The FDA only approves herbs for use in food, not in cosmetics, but that doesn't mean they aren't safe to use as coloring agents, just that they must be used in the soap for the herbal properties they impart.) Some common herbs for coloring soap include turmeric (yellow), nettle (green), annatto (yellow or orange), alkanet root (purple), and indigo (blue). To use herbs to color your soap, grind them finely and add them directly to your soap or lye-water, or infuse them into the oils in the recipe. Many herbs lose their color when mixed with sodium hydroxide; over time, some herb-based colors will fade from finished soap.

Clay is another all-natural material for coloring soap. It is mined from the earth and is basically finely ground rock. Because clay absorbs water, it is essential to premix it with water before adding it to the soap mixture to ensure your soap does not dry out and crack. Only use cosmetic-grade clays; pottery clays often are not held to the same standards as cosmetic clays and may contaminate your soap.

Adding Fragrance

Fragrance provides another way for you to show your personal preferences, style, and point of view in your soapmaking. You can choose scents to match your design or to match your personal ethos. Many ingredients can add fragrance to soap, but the two that work best are fragrance oils and essential oils. Other ingredients — infused oils, extracts, and perfumes — are not recommended for scenting soap.

Using Fragrance Oils

Fragrance oils are synthetic blends of aroma chemicals and essential oils (discussed further below). Most fine perfumes and colognes are created with fragrance oils. A fragrance may have up to 300 different ingredients to achieve a desired scent profile. Fragrance oils go through rigorous testing to ensure that they are safe.

Fragrance oils are the most widely used material for adding scent to products because of their wide range of scents, their safety record, and their batch-to-batch consistency. Some scents can only be found as fragrance oils, including chocolate and strawberry, neither of which can be made naturally.

Because fragrance oils are a mixture of many synthetic aroma chemicals, they are the most frequent cause of batch failure in cold-process soaping. Soapmakers can mitigate this risk by using fragrances that have been fully tested by the manufacturer to ensure that they work in cold-process soapmaking, smell strong, and have staying power in the finished soap.

Fragrance oils are typically added at thin trace. Some fragrance oils, especially vanilla-based ones, contain natural discoloring agents. Thus, most fragrances with sweeter notes of vanilla, baking notes, caramel, or chocolate will often discolor soap brown. Other fragrances may discolor soap a light yellow, or more rarely, a light purple or pink.

Using Essential Oils for Fragrance

Essential oils are volatile organic compounds that offer an all-natural method of scenting soap. They are extracted from parts of plants: tree bark, the leaves of shrubs, flower petals, and so on. There are a variety of ways to extract essential oils. Nonchemical methods include steam distillation, enfleurage, pressing, and expressing. Chemical methods include solvent extraction and CO_2 (carbon dioxide) extraction.

Fragrancing Precautions

Both fragrance oils and essential oils must be treated with care. Always store them in their original bottles and use glass or stainless steel mixing bowls and stirring utensils when working with them. They can degrade rubber and plastic or even eat holes in softer materials. Be aware that fragrance oils and essential oils may damage work surfaces and ruin nail polish.

Essential oils have some particular safety guidelines. Undiluted essential oils can irritate skin and mucous membranes, so as with other soaping steps, work in a well-ventilated space when mixing them. Gloves may be warranted.

If you choose to experiment with essential oils not used in this book, please research their properties carefully before incorporating them into your soap. If you are pregnant, please consult with your doctor about making and using soap with essential oils.

Essential oils have been used for centuries to fragrance products and for their many beneficial properties. Pure essential oils are purported to have calming and mood-stabilizing effects, to heal and soothe many physical ailments, and to promote overall health. While the FDA makes no therapeutic or medical claims about essential oils, it sees no danger in using them to scent your soap and body products.

Like fragrance oils, there are guidelines for essential oils regarding how to much to use, which are safe to use on the body versus the face, and which irritate skin. Because oils are derived from plants and harvested annually, their scent and potency can vary from year to year depending on growing conditions. The method of extraction or distillation can also affect essential oils' smell.

Essential oils can be extremely delicate in the high-pH environment of soapmaking. Not all essential oils will last in cold-process soap. For example, regular orange essential oil withers in the harsh raw-soap environment. To achieve a scent of orange, you need to use an oil that has been distilled a number of times to concentrate the aroma molecules. These are labeled orange 5× or orange 10×, depending on how many distillations have occurred.

Essential oils are typically added during thin trace. Some essential oils will imbue the soap with their own colors, generally light yellow to bright orange to green. It's easy to work with the colors to turn them into part of your design.

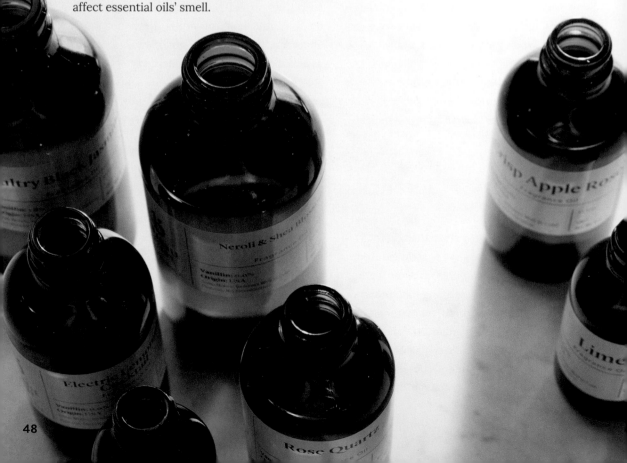

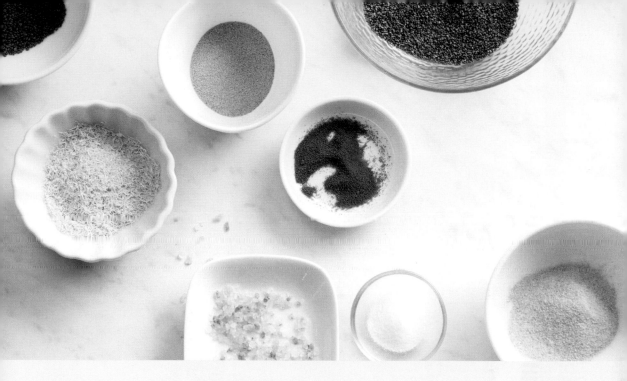

Adding Exfoliants to Soap

Popular exfoliants for cold-process soap include colloidal oatmeal, bamboo extract powder, pumice, walnut shells, ground pumpkin seeds, crushed grape seeds, jojoba beads, flaxseeds, chia seeds, salts and sugars, shredded or sliced loofah, poppy seeds, coffee grounds, cranberry seeds, strawberry seeds, and others.

Consider the following points when choosing additives for your soap.

1 Additives can be very scratchy and rough on skin depending on their size and shape; a good starting amount is 1 teaspoon (5 mL) of additive per pound (454 g) of soap. What might feel harsh and scratchy on your skin may be perfect for another person or another body part.

The key to finding the right scrubby additive for your project is to test, test, test. Make a small test batch with a new exfoliant and ask friends and family for input about how your product feels. You can always add more to the next batch, but you can't take it out once it's in.

2 Always buy food-grade or cosmetic-grade additives. Make sure food-grade seeds have been irradiated so they cannot sprout. In a moist environment, like the shower, live seeds could very well turn into little plants!

3 Some additives, like ground flaxseeds, clays, and chia seeds, absorb liquid. For these additives, mix each teaspoon (5 mL) of the additive in 1 tablespoon (15 mL) of water before adding it to the soap batter. If you add a water-absorbing additive to your soap without doing this, the soap could dry too quickly, causing cracking.

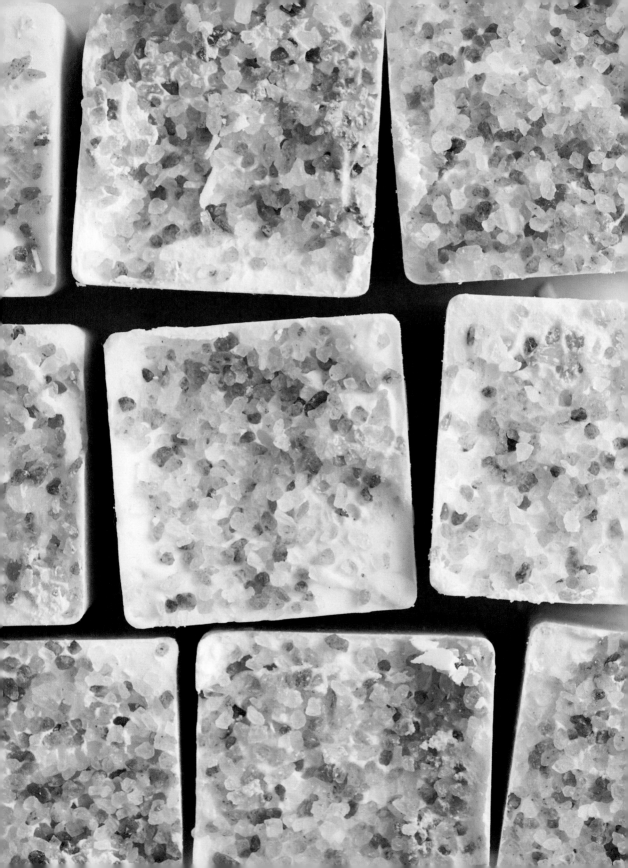

CHAPTER FIVE

Recipes

●●● — ● — ●●●

These recipes are listed by the complexity of the techniques, from beginner to intermediate to advanced. As mentioned previously, working with milk presents some challenges, so I urge you to become familiar with the basics of making soap with water before you try using milk as an ingredient. Once you have some experience, I know you'll enjoy experimenting with both mammal and plant-based milks.

To show the range of options, I've chosen specific milks for many of these recipes, but you can substitute any milk in any recipe on a one-to-one basis. For example, if a recipe calls for 6.5 ounces of sour cream, use 6.5 ounces of milk, yogurt, nut milk, or whatever milk you want to experiment with. Note that in some of the recipes, milk replaces the full amount of water to be mixed with lye; those are marked "100% replacement." Many of them use primarily water

to mix with lye, but call for a certain amount of the water to be replaced with milk and added at trace; those are marked with the percentage of water that is being replaced, for example "30% added at trace."

A final note: Many of these recipes are made with fragrance oils, but if you prefer to substitute essential oils, I've included suggestions. Some of the usage rates are different, so follow the instructions for each recipe.

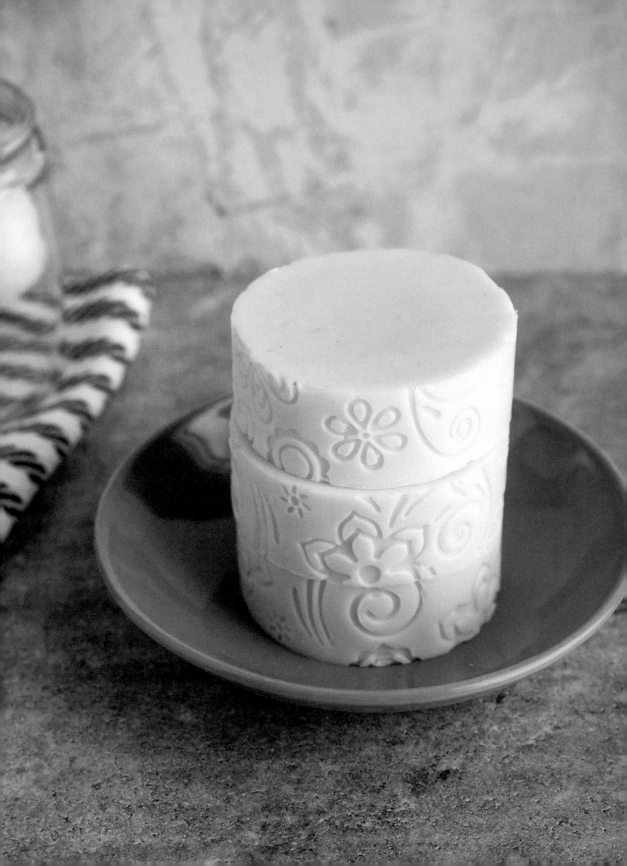

Shea and Aloe Bars
with Yogurt

30% ADDED AT TRACE • MAKES 8 BARS

This elegant, skin-nourishing soap contains soothing aloe vera as well as whole-milk yogurt and a heaping helping of shea butter for extra creaminess. The simple technique utilizes a texture mat to produce an interesting and sophisticated design. Homemade yogurt is the best; if you prefer to buy it, use plain yogurt and choose a brand with as few additives as possible.

Mold and Special Tools

Silicone column mold
Texture mat

Oil Amounts

6.0 ounces/170 g
coconut oil (25%)
3.6 ounces/102 g
babassu oil (15%)
3.6 ounces/102 g
hazelnut seed oil (15%)
3.6 ounces/102 g
shea butter (15%)
3.6 ounces/102 g
sunflower seed oil (15%)
2.4 ounces/68 g
pure olive oil (10%)

1.2 ounces/34 g
castor oil (5%)

Lye-Water

3.6 ounces/102 g
distilled water
3.4 ounces/96 g
lye (6% superfat)
2 teaspoons/10 mL
sodium lactate

Fragrance Oil

1.7 ounces/48 g
White Tea and Ginger

Essential Oil Alternative
1.2 ounces/34 g
ylang ylang

Colorant

1 teaspoon/5 mL
titanium dioxide
dispersed into
1 tablespoon/15 mL
sunflower seed oil

Additives

2.3 ounces/65 g
yogurt
2.0 ounces/57 g
aloe vera

Safe Soaping!

Wear proper safety gear the whole time · Work in a well-ventilated space · No distractions

Use Any Milk

As with all these recipes, you can substitute any other kind of milk or dairy product, used in the same amount.

Prepare Ahead

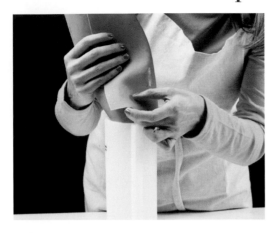

1 Roll up the texture mat and insert it into the assembled column mold.

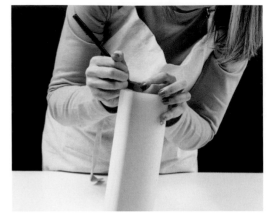

2 Mark the mat for cutting. You want the edges to line up inside the mold without overlapping.

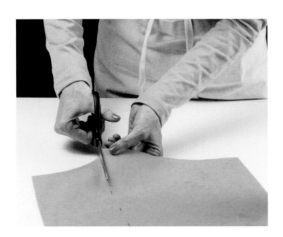

3 Cut the mat to fit.

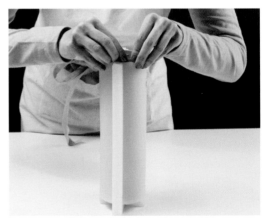

4 Unroll the mat inside the mold and press it into place.

Make the Soap Batter

1 Melt the babassu oil in its original container and measure it into a heatproof bowl large enough to hold the entire recipe. Melt and measure the coconut oil and add it to the bowl. Add the shea butter to the hot oils and stir until melted. If needed, microwave the bowl in 15-second bursts to melt the shea butter completely. Add the hazelnut oil, sunflower seed oil, olive oil, and castor oil and set the bowl aside.

2 Measure the distilled water and the lye into separate heatproof containers. Add the lye to the water a tablespoon (15 mL) at a time (never add the liquid to the lye). Stir continuously until the lye fully dissolves and the water becomes clear. Stir the sodium lactate into the lye-water.

3 When the oils and the lye-water have cooled to about 105°F (40.5°C), add the lye-water to the oils, pouring it over the shaft of the stick blender to minimize air bubbles.

4 Insert the stick blender into the batter, tilting it so that any trapped air can escape. *Do not turn on the stick blender until the blades are fully immersed.* Alternate pulsing and stirring with the stick blender until a thin trace is achieved.

Mix and Pour

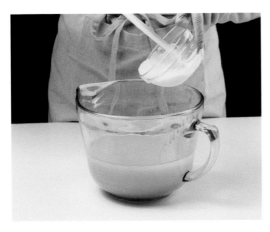

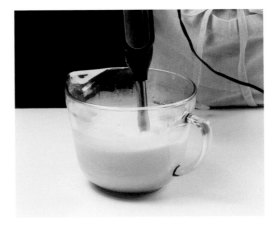

5 Add the yogurt, aloe vera, fragrance oil, and titanium dioxide to the soap batter.

6 Blend until just combined and pour into the mold.

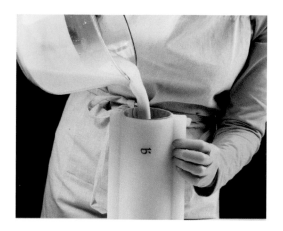

Final Steps

Let sit at room temperature for at least 48 hours before unmolding.

Gently peel the liner away from the soap; if it sticks, wait another 24 hours.

Cut into bars using a knife. Let the bars cure in a well-ventilated area for 4 to 6 weeks before using, turning them every few days so that they cure evenly.

7 Pour before the batter gets too thick so it can flow into the crevices in the texture mat and pick up all the details in the design.

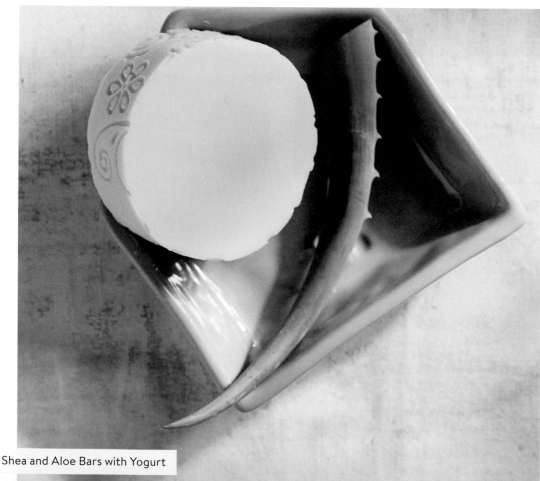

Calendula-Infused
Buttermilk Bars

50% ADDED AT TRACE • MAKES 10 BARS

This all-natural buttermilk recipe is packed with skin-loving calendula as an extract and an oil infusion and sprinkled with petals for added exfoliating power. Kokum butter and palm kernel flakes thicken the batter for flat layering and top texturing. Homemade buttermilk is best; if you buy it, use a brand with as few additives as possible.

The recipe is formulated using sunflower oil to infuse the calendula; using a commercial calendula-infused oil will change the results. If you do use a commercial product, run the ingredients list through a lye calculator to make sure it will work.

This essential oil produces a softly fragranced soap; for a stronger scent, substitute the same amount of Pink Grapefruit fragrance oil. These bars go in the freezer overnight to prevent overheating.

Mold and Special Tools

Tall 12-inch (30.5 cm) silicone loaf mold
Easy-pour container
Double boiler (or a small pot nested in a larger one)

Oil Amounts

8.7 ounces/247 g coconut oil (25%)
8.7 ounces/247 g palm oil (25%)
5.2 ounces/147 g pure olive oil (15%)
3.5 ounces/99 g kokum butter (10%)
3.5 ounces/99 g palm kernel flakes (10%)
3.5 ounces/99 g calendula-infused sunflower seed oil (10%)
1.7 ounces/48 g castor oil (5%)

Lye-Water

5.7 ounces/162 g distilled water
5.0 ounces/142 g lye (5% superfat)
3 teaspoons/15 mL sodium lactate

Essential Oil

2.5 ounces/71 g grapefruit

Colorant

1 teaspoon/5 mL yellow oxide dispersed into 1 tablespoon/15 mL sunflower seed oil

Additives

5.7 ounces/162 g buttermilk
4 tablespoons/60 mL dried calendula petals, divided
1.5 ounces/43 g calendula extract

Safe Soaping!

Wear proper safety gear the whole time · Work in a well-ventilated space · No distractions

Use Any Milk

As with all these recipes, you can substitute any other kind of milk or dairy product, used in the same amount.

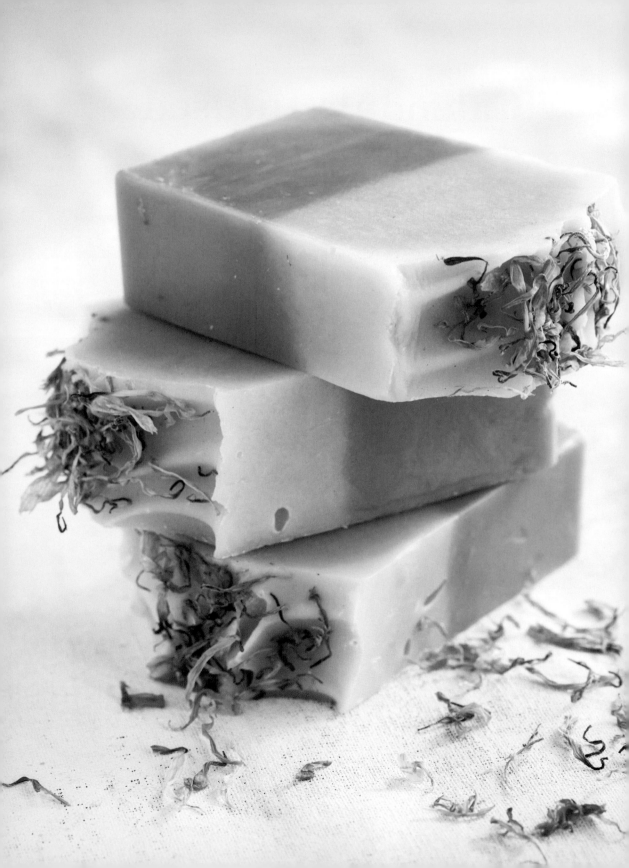

Prepare Ahead

To make the calendula-infused oil, put 2 tablespoons of the calendula petals in the double boiler. Pour 4.0 ounces (113 g) of sunflower seed oil on top of the petals. (You need to infuse a little extra oil, as some is absorbed.) Heat on medium-low for 4 to 6 hours, stirring occasionally. Remove from the heat, let cool, and strain out the petals.

Measure out the buttermilk and bring to room temperature.

Make the Soap Batter

1 Melt the palm oil in its original container, mix it thoroughly, and measure it into a heatproof bowl large enough to hold the entire recipe. Melt and measure the coconut oil and add it to the bowl. Add the kokum butter and palm kernel flakes to the hot oils and stir until melted. If needed, microwave the bowl in 10-second bursts to melt the butter completely. Add the olive oil, infused sunflower seed oil, and castor oil and set the bowl aside.

2 Measure the distilled water and the lye into separate heatproof containers. Add the lye to the water a tablespoon (15 mL) at a time (never add the liquid to the lye). Stir continuously until the lye fully dissolves and the water becomes clear. Stir the sodium lactate into the lye-water.

3 When the oils and the lye-water have cooled to about 105°F (40.5°C), add the lye-water to the oils, pouring it over the shaft of the stick blender to minimize air bubbles.

4 Insert the stick blender into the batter, tilting it so that any trapped air can escape. *Do not turn on the stick blender until the blades are fully immersed.* Alternate pulsing and stirring with the stick blender until a thin trace is achieved.

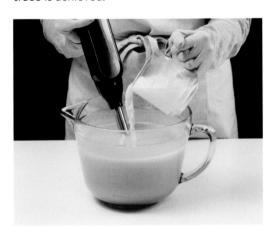

5 Add the buttermilk, grapefruit essential oil, and calendula extract. Stick-blend until combined and you achieve a medium/thin trace.

Color and Pour

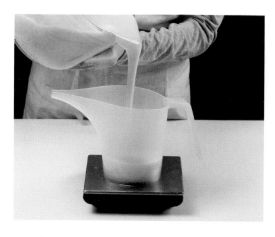

7 Pour half the batter (about 26 ounces/ 737 g) into an easy-pour container and set aside.

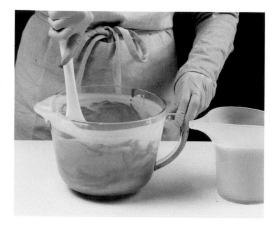

8 Add 1 teaspoon (5 mL) of dispersed yellow oxide to the remaining batter and mix it in with a spatula.

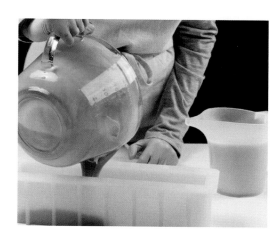

9 Once the color is fully mixed in and the batter is thick enough to support layers, pour the yellow batter into the mold.

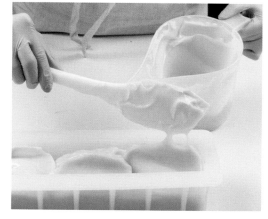

10 If your white batter is too thin, stick-blend a bit more to achieve a medium trace. Gently pour or spoon the plain batter on top of the yellow. Work low and slow, being careful to create layers without breaking through.

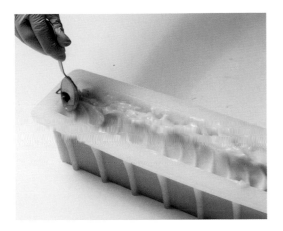

11 Texture the top with a spoon by pushing the batter up from the longer sides toward the center to create a peak down the center of the loaf.

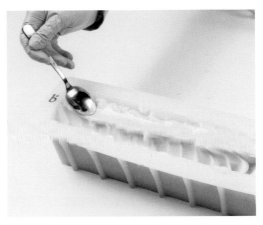

12 Run the back of the spoon down the center of the peak to flatten it out.

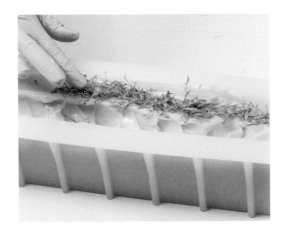

13 Sprinkle the remaining calendula petals down the center of the mold, where the soap is highest. Press very slightly with a gloved finger to help it stick without damaging the texture.

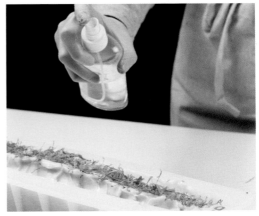

14 Spray thoroughly with 99% rubbing alcohol to prevent soda ash.

Final Steps

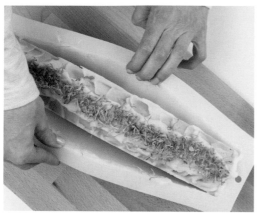

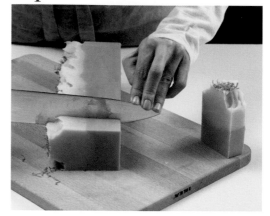

15 Buttermilk will heat up and partially gel if left at room temperature. Avoid this by placing the soap in the freezer overnight. Remove from the freezer and wait at least 48 hours to unmold. Frozen soaps tend to soften quite a bit as they thaw and need time to harden again.

16 To slice the bars, lay the loaf on its side and cut with a knife. This prevents the herbs from being pulled through the soap and leaving drag marks. It also keeps the textured top from being damaged while cutting.

Let the bars cure in a well-ventilated area for 4 to 6 weeks before using, turning them every few days to ensure they cure evenly.

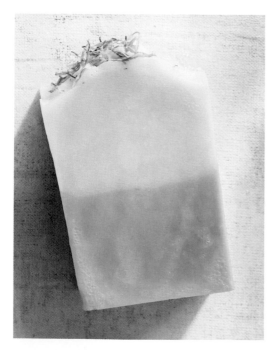

Textured Rose Clay Bars
with Nonfat Milk

100% REPLACEMENT • MAKES 12 BARS

This nourishing recipe creates simple and elegant bars of soap. With a generous amount of shea butter, rose clay, and evening primrose extract, the final product is nourishing and conditioning for skin. Nonfat milk has slightly more lactose than whole milk, but the lower fat content leads to fluffier bubbles and a slightly harder bar. A dusting of light gold mica on the textured tops gives these otherwise plain bars a delicate shimmer.

Mold and Special Tools

12-cavity rectangular silicone mold
Fine-mesh strainer
Fork
Powder sprayer filled with light gold mica
Cutting board for moving mold to freezer

Oil Amounts

13.5 ounces/383 g pure olive oil (30%)
11.7 ounces/332 g coconut oil (26%)
11.25 ounces/319 g palm oil (25%)

6.75 ounces/191 g shea butter (15%)
1.8 ounces/51 g castor oil (4%)

Lye Mixture

13.2 ounces/374 g nonfat milk, frozen
6.3 ounces/179 g lye (4% superfat)
4 teaspoons/20 mL sodium lactate

Fragrance Oil

3.3 ounces/94 g Rose Quartz

Essential Oil Alternative

1 ounce/28 g peppermint 2nd distilled
2.1 ounces/60 g red Brazilian mandarin

Colorant

4 teaspoons/20 mL rose clay dispersed into
1½ tablespoons/22.5 mL distilled water
Light Gold mica

Additive

1 ounce/28 g evening primrose extract

Safe Soaping!

Wear proper safety gear the whole time · Work in a well-ventilated space · No distractions

Use Any Milk

As with all these recipes, you can substitute any other kind of milk or dairy product, used in the same amount.

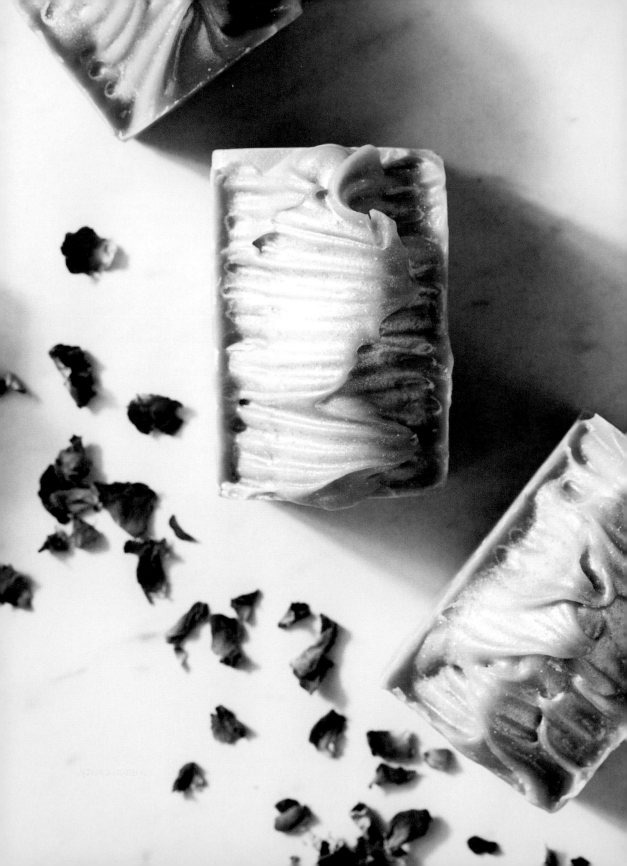

Make the Soap Batter

1 Melt the palm oil in its original container, mix it thoroughly, and measure it into a heatproof bowl large enough to hold the entire recipe. Melt and measure the coconut oil and add it to the bowl. Add the shea butter to the hot oils and stir until melted. If needed, microwave the bowl in 10-second bursts to melt the butter completely. Add the olive oil and castor oil and set the bowl aside.

2 Measure the frozen milk and the lye into separate heatproof containers. Slowly add the lye to the milk a tablespoon (15 mL) at a time, stirring continuously until all the lye has fully dissolved. This can take up to 30 minutes due to the cold temperature. Add the sodium lactate to the lye mixture and stir to combine.

3 When the oils have cooled to between 100 and 105°F (38–40.5°C) and the lye mixture is between 75 and 85°F (24–29°C), gently pour the lye mixture through the strainer into the oils, stirring any residue gently with a spatula.

4 Insert the stick blender into the batter, tilting it so that any trapped air can escape. *Do not turn on the stick blender until the blades are fully immersed.* Alternate pulsing and stirring with the stick blender until a thin trace is achieved.

Color and Pour

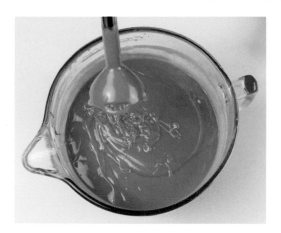

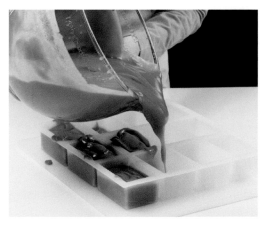

5 Add the evening primrose extract, fragrance oil, and dispersed rose clay and whisk to combine. Stick-blend until medium/thick trace.

6 Place the mold on top of the cutting board. Pour the batter into the molds. It may not all fit at first, but as the batter thickens, you will be able to spoon more into each cavity.

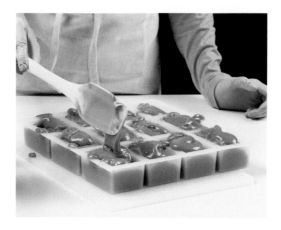

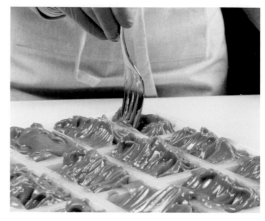

7 Give the batter a couple minutes to thicken if needed and then add more batter to each bar with a spoon or spatula to create a mound.

8 Texture the tops of the bars by pushing the batter up and toward the center of each bar with a fork; try to create a wavelike shape in the middle of each bar. Wipe the fork clean with a paper towel when necessary.

9 Place the light gold mica into the powder duster and gently tap it over the soap to lightly dust the surface.

Final Steps

This is a rare recipe where spraying with alcohol will damage the mica on the surface. If the bars do develop ash on top, you can remove it with a small, handheld clothes steamer. Move the mold into the freezer and let sit overnight.

Remove from the freezer and unmold immediately. (Freezing makes it easier to remove the textured bars from the silicone mold.)

Frozen soaps tend to soften quite a bit as they thaw and need time to harden again.

Let the bars cure in a well-ventilated area for 4 to 6 weeks before using, turning them every few days to ensure they cure evenly.

Exfoliating Lemon Bars
with Coconut Milk

30% ADDED AT TRACE • MAKES 6 BARS

Soaping with coconut milk can be tricky because the additional sugars can cause the soap to overheat, resulting in cracking or uneven texture in the bars, and the batter may sometimes overflow the molds. For this recipe, use the freezer to prevent overheating. These bars fit perfectly into your hand, and the lemon peel powder provides gentle exfoliation. This recipe's higher superfat compensates for the extra cleansing ability of the coconut oil.

Molds
6 half-cylinder silicone molds

Oil Amount
20 ounces/567 g
   coconut oil (100%)

Lye-Water
3.5 ounces/100 g
   distilled water
2.8 ounces/80 g
   lye (20% superfat)
1 teaspoon/5 mL
   sodium lactate

Fragrance Oil Blend
0.7 ounce/20 g
   Coconut Cream
0.7 ounce/20 g
   Sweet Meyer Lemon

Essential Oil Alternative
1.4 ounces/40 g lemon

Additives
2 teaspoons/10 mL
   lemon peel powder
2.3 ounces/65 g
   canned coconut milk

Safe Soaping!
Wear proper safety gear the whole time · Work in a well-ventilated space · No distractions

Use Any Milk
As with all these recipes, you can substitute any other kind of milk or dairy product, used in the same amount.

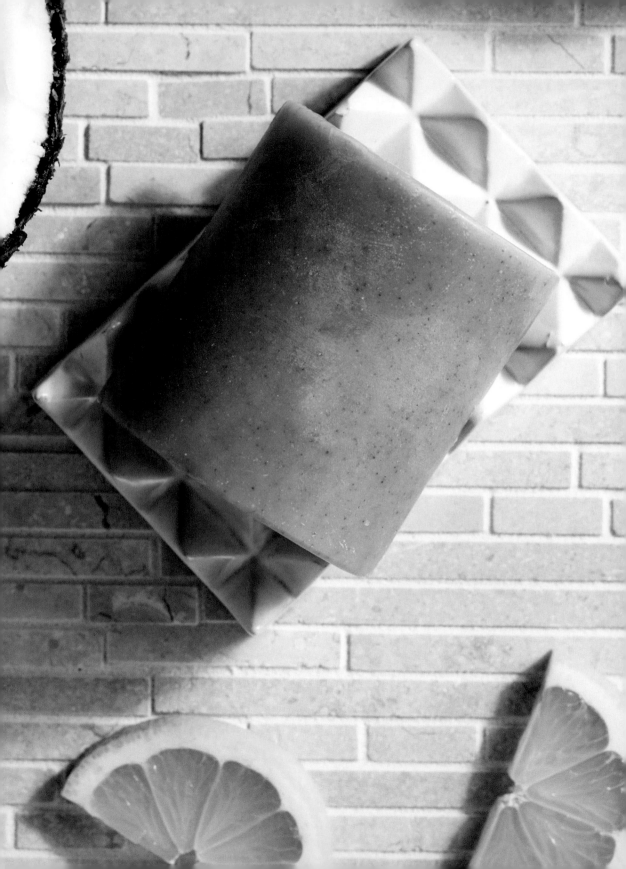

Prepare Ahead

Shake the can of coconut milk to thoroughly mix. Measure the coconut milk and keep in the refrigerator until ready to start soaping.

Make the Soap Batter

1 Melt the coconut oil in Its original container and measure It into a heatproof bowl large enough to hold the entire recipe with room to mix. Measure the distilled water and the lye into separate heatproof containers. Add the lye to the water a tablespoon (15 mL) at a time (never add the liquid to the lye). Stir continuously until the lye fully dissolves and the water becomes clear. Stir the sodium lactate into the lye-water.

2 When the oil and the lye-water have cooled to about 105°F (40.5°C), add the lye-water to the oil, pouring it over the shaft of the stick blender to minimize air bubbles.

3 Insert the stick blender into the batter, tilting it so that any trapped air can escape. *Do not turn on the stick blender until the blades are fully immersed.* Alternate pulsing and stirring with the stick blender until you reach emulsion.

Mix and Pour

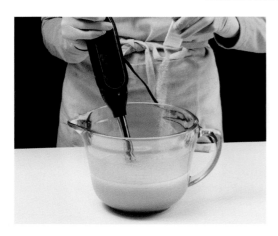

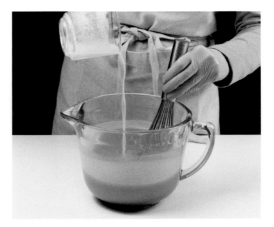

4 Add the fragrance oils and lemon peel powder. Stick-blend to combine and break up any clumps. The batter should be at thin trace.

5 Add the coconut milk and whisk by hand until fully mixed in. (Mix quickly, as the coconut milk will thicken and heat up the batter.)

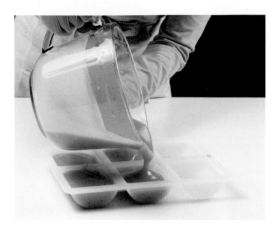

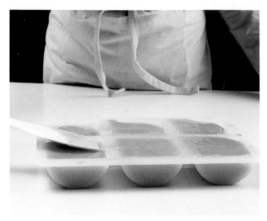

6 Pour or spoon the batter into the molds.

7 Use a spatula to flatten the tops of the soaps.

Final Steps

Spray thoroughly with 99% rubbing alcohol to prevent soda ash. Place the molds in the freezer overnight to avoid overheating.

Remove from the freezer and wait 48 hours before unmolding. Frozen soaps tend to soften quite a bit as they thaw and need time to harden again.

Let the bars cure in a well-ventilated area for 4 to 6 weeks before using, turning them every few days to ensure they cure evenly.

Layered Clay
and Oat Milk Bars

50% ADDED AT TRACE · MAKES 3–4 BARS

This palm-free recipe uses pure and natural clays for color. The batch contains a full 50 percent oat milk with oat extract. (The oat milk is added at the end because lye added to oat milk makes a sticky, clumpy, stringy mess.) Ginger essential oil accelerates the soap batter and clay thickens it, making it easier to pour straight, even layers. Starting with a thin trace and stirring by hand afterward are recommended.

Mold and Special Tools

4-inch (10 cm) silicone loaf mold
Spoon for texturing top
4 easy-pour containers
Soap beveller (optional)

Oil Amounts

4.2 ounces/119 g
coconut oil (30%)
2.8 ounces/80 g
sweet almond oil (20%)
2.8 ounces/80 g
rice bran oil (20%)
1.4 ounces/40 g
mango butter (10%)
1.4 ounces/40 g
macadamia nut oil (10%)
0.7 ounce/20 g
avocado butter (5%)
0.7 ounce/20 g
castor oil (5%)

Lye-Water

2.3 ounces/65 g
distilled water
2.0 ounces/57 g
lye (2% superfat)
1 teaspoon/5 mL
sodium lactate

Essential Oil Blend

0.4 ounce/11 g
ginger
0.5 ounce/14 g
Valencia orange

Colorants

Disperse the first three into 1 tablespoon/15 mL distilled water each.

1 teaspoon/5 mL
yellow Brazilian clay
1 teaspoon/5 mL
dark red Brazilian clay
1 teaspoon/5 mL
green zeolite clay
1 teaspoon/5 mL
indigo powder dispersed into 1 tablespoon/15 mL sweet almond oil

Additives

2.3 ounces/65 g
oat milk (see page 10)
0.5 ounce/14 g
oat extract

Safe Soaping!

Wear proper safety gear the whole time · Work in a well-ventilated space · No distractions

Use Any Milk

As with all these recipes, you can substitute any other kind of milk or dairy product, used in the same amount.

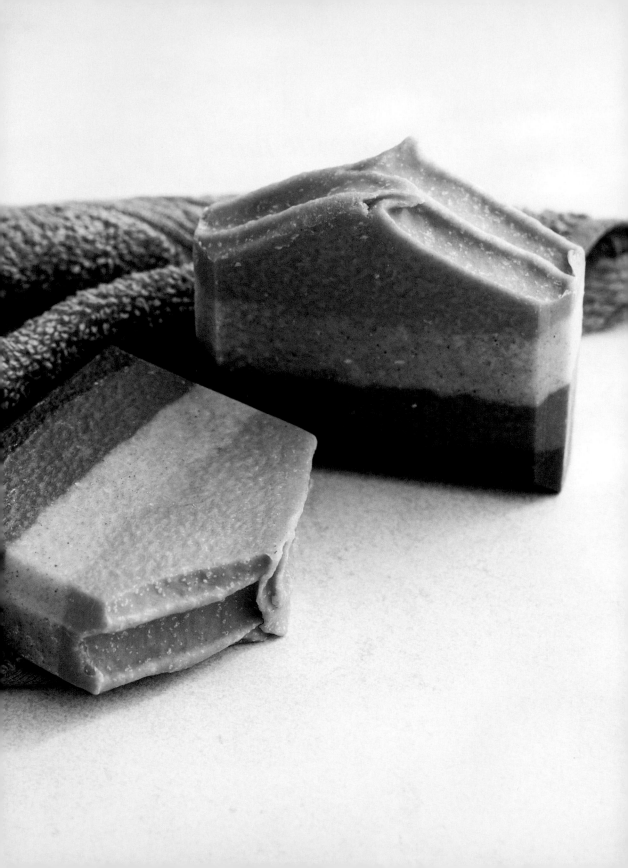

Make the Soap Batter

1 Melt and measure the coconut oil into a heatproof bowl large enough to hold the entire recipe. Add the avocado butter and mango butter to the hot coconut oil and stir until melted. If needed, microwave the bowl in 10-second bursts to melt the butter completely. Add the sweet almond oil, rice bran oil, macadamia nut oil, and castor oil and set the bowl aside.

2 Measure the distilled water and the lye into separate heatproof containers. Add the lye to the water a tablespoon (15 mL) at a time (never add the liquid to the lye). Stir continuously until the lye fully dissolves and the water becomes clear. Stir the sodium lactate into the lye-water.

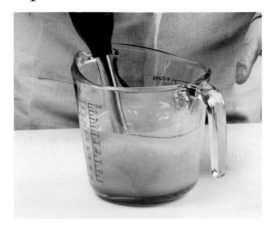

4 Insert the stick blender into the batter, tilting it so that any trapped air can escape. *Do not turn on the stick blender until the blades are fully immersed.* Alternate pulsing and stirring with the stick blender until a very thin trace is achieved.

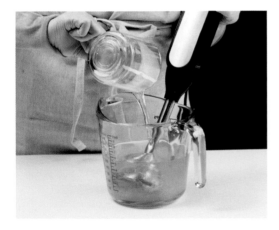

3 When the oils and the lye-water have cooled to about 105°F (40.5°C), add the lye-water to the oils, pouring it over the shaft of the stick blender to minimize air bubbles.

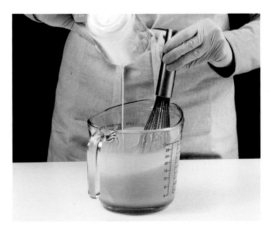

5 Add the oat extract and oat milk and stir with a whisk to incorporate.

Color and Pour

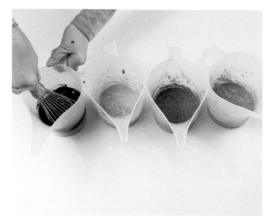

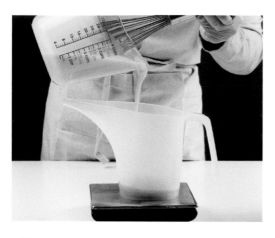

6 Divide the batter equally among the easy-pour containers (a little more than 5 ounces/142 g each).

7 Add the clays and the the indigo to the containers, one color per container, and whisk from lightest to darkest to combine.

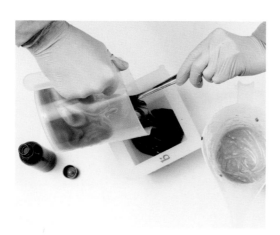

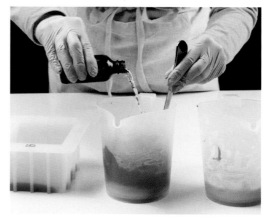

8 Add about ¼ of the essential oil blend into the indigo batter and mix well by hand. Pour all of the indigo batter into the mold, tapping it on the counter to smooth out the layer.

9 Add another ¼ of the essential oil blend to the red batter (eyeballing it is fine!) and mix well by hand.

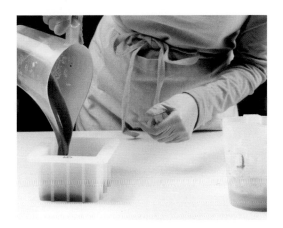

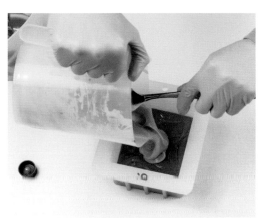

10 Pour all of the red batter low and slow over the indigo, tapping the mold or smoothing the batter with your spatula to make an even layer.

11 Repeat with the green batter, then with the yellow, adding half of the remaining essential oil blend to each color and again pouring low onto the previous batter. You may need to use a spoon or spatula at this point to smooth out the last layer.

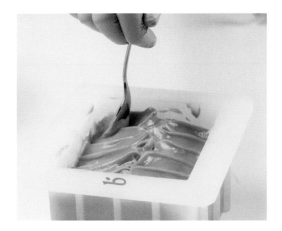

12 Use the spoon to create texture on top of the batter. We used the spoon's tip to drag batter from the outer edges of the mold up and in, creating waves leading to the center and a taller peak in the middle.

Final Steps

Spray thoroughly with 99% rubbing alcohol several times over 90 minutes to prevent soda ash. Let the mold sit at room temperature for 48 hours before you unmold the soap. Slice the loaf into bars and bevel the edges, if desired.

Let the bars cure in a well-ventilated area for 4 to 6 weeks before using, turning them every few days to ensure they cure evenly.

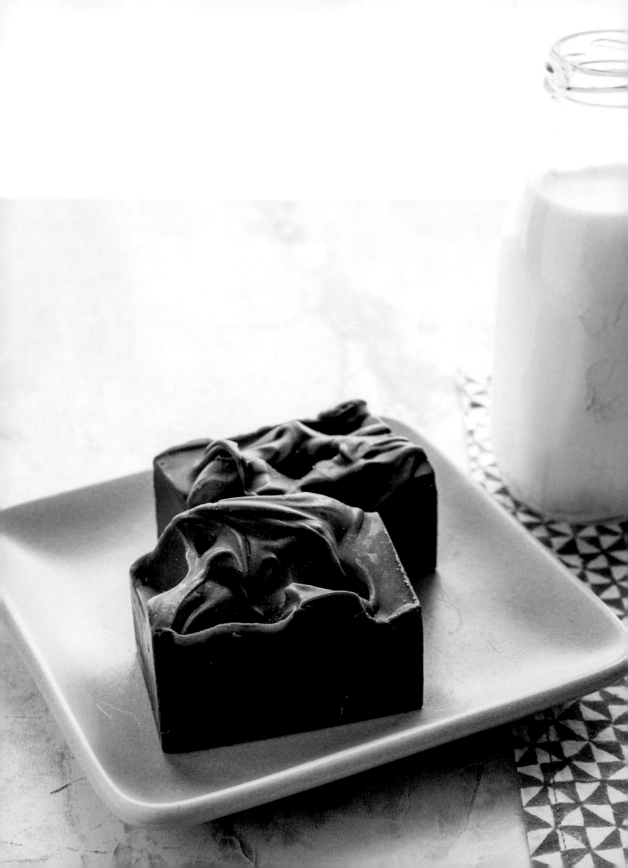

Charcoal Facial Bars
with Whole Milk and Aloe

100% REPLACEMENT • MAKES 9 BARS

Black soap? Seriously? Don't worry — this soap is designed to be a fantastic facial cleansing bar. The charcoal adds dramatic color, but it lathers up clean. This all-natural, palm-free recipe is based on one of the most popular recipes on the Soap Queen blog. It's formulated with luxurious oils and delicately scented with lavender and tea tree.

Mold and Special Tools

9-bar birchwood mold
   with silicone liner
Dividers for mold
Spoon for texturing tops
Fine-mesh strainer

Oil Amounts

9.9 ounces/281 g
   olive pomace oil (30%)
6.6 ounces/187 g
   coconut oil (20%)
4.9 ounces/139 g
   shea butter (15%)
3.3 ounces/94 g
   mango butter (10%)

3.3 ounces/94 g
   jojoba oil (10%)
1.6 ounces/45 g
   argan oil (5%)
1.6 ounces/45 g
   tamanu oil (5%)
1.6 ounces/45 g
   castor oil (5%)

Lye Mixture

10.8 ounces/306 g
   whole milk, frozen
4.3 ounces/122 g
   lye (5% superfat)
3 teaspoons/15 mL
   sodium lactate

Essential Oil Blend

1.2 ounces/34 g
   lavender 40/42
1.2 ounces/34 g
   tea tree

Colorant

4 teaspoons/20 mL
   activated charcoal

Additive

1.5 ounces/43 g
   aloe extract

Safe Soaping!

Wear proper safety gear the whole time · Work in a well-ventilated space · No distractions

Use Any Milk

As with all these recipes, you can substitute any other kind of milk or dairy product, used in the same amount.

Prepare Ahead

Place the silicone liner into the birchwood mold. Assemble the dividers and place them nearby, but not in the mold.

Make the Soap Batter

1 Melt and measure the coconut oil into a heatproof bowl large enough to hold the entire recipe. Add the shea butter and mango butter to the hot coconut oil and stir until melted. If needed, microwave the bowl in 10-second bursts to melt the butter completely. Add the argan oil, jojoba oil, olive pomace oil, tamanu oil, and castor oil and set the bowl aside.

2 Measure the frozen milk and the lye into separate heatproof containers. Slowly add the lye to the milk a tablespoon (15 mL) at a time, stirring continuously until all the lye has fully dissolved. This can take up to 30 minutes due to the cold temperature.

Add the sodium lactate to the lye mixture and stir to combine.

3 When the oils have cooled to between 100 and 105°F (38–40.5°C) and the lye mixture is between 75 and 85°F (24–29°C), gently pour the lye mixture through the strainer into the oils, stirring any residue gently with a spatula.

4 Insert the stick blender into the batter, tilting it so that any trapped air can escape. *Do not turn on the stick blender until the blades are fully immersed.* Alternate pulsing and stirring with the stick blender until a thin trace is achieved.

Mix and Pour

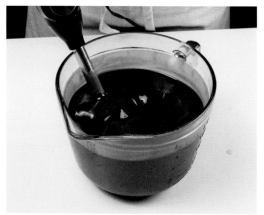

5 Add the aloe extract, essential oil blend, and charcoal. Charcoal is very lightweight, so before you turn on the stick blender, push the powder under the surface to keep it from puffing up out of the bowl. Once the charcoal is mixed in, stick-blend to medium/thick trace. It needs to be pretty thick to create the right texture.

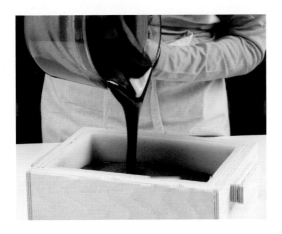

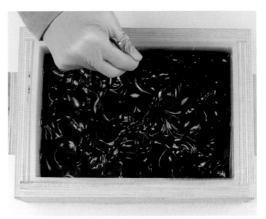

6 Pour or spoon the batter into the mold. If the batter is too thin to texture right away, let it sit in the mold until it thickens, checking it every minute or two.

7 Texture the top of the batter with a spoon. We used little dabbing/swirling motions with the back of a spoon to create this look, but have fun with this step and create whatever texture you like.

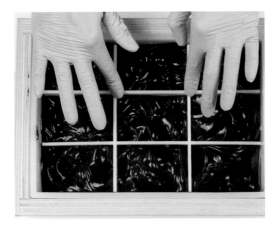

Final Steps

Spray thoroughly with 99% rubbing alcohol several times over 90 minutes to prevent soda ash. Let the soap sit at room temperature for at least 48 hours before unmolding.

Let the bars cure in a well-ventilated area for 4 to 6 weeks before using, turning them every few days to ensure they cure evenly.

TECHNIQUE TIP

Use sliding or twisting motions to separate the soaps from the dividers. Pulling the dividers directly away from the bars will tear them and leave jagged sides.

8 Insert the dividers into the soap. If this disrupts the texturing, use the spoon to retexture the individual bars.

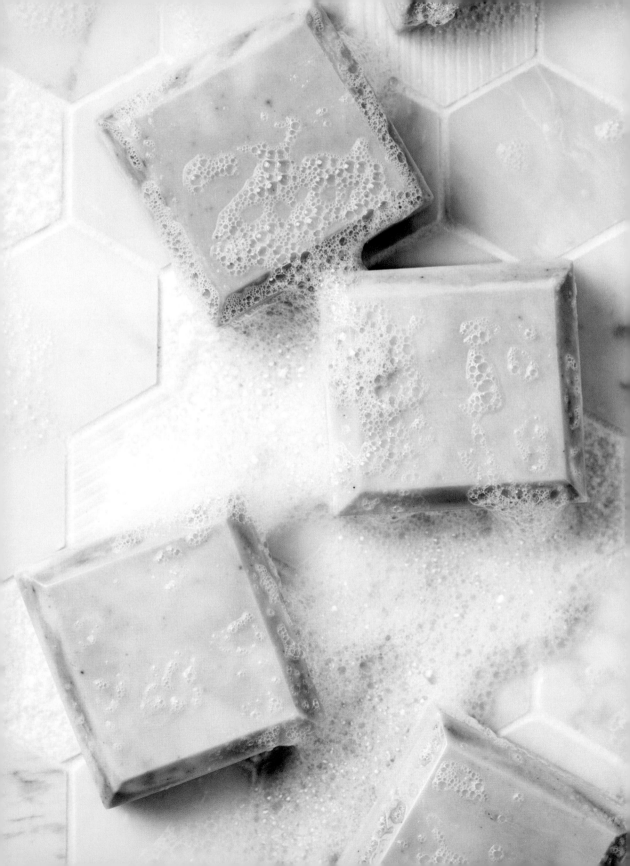

In-the-Pot
Swirl Buttermilk Castile

50% ADDED AT TRACE • MAKES 12 BARS

This gentle recipe is made with 100 percent olive oil, making it a true castile bar (made famous in Spain and prized for its kindness to sensitive skin). Homemade buttermilk is best; if you buy it, use a brand with as few additives as possible. The colorant comes from dried madder root, a climbing plant with pale yellow flowers. The lavender-and-peppermint essential oil blend smells amazing. The soap is designed with an in-the-pot swirl and finished with beveled edges.

This mold is large and flexible, so a cutting board placed under it will be handy if you need to move the soaps after pouring. The bars need extra cure and hardening time thanks to the large amount of olive oil in the recipe.

Mold and Special Tools

12-bar square silicone mold
Cutting board for moving
    the mold
2 large bowls
Soap beveller (optional)

Oil Amount

40 ounces/1,134 g
    pure olive oil (100%)

Lye-Mixture

6.6 ounces/187 g
    distilled water
5.2 ounces lye (3% superfat)
1 tablespoon/15 mL
    sodium lactate

Essential Oil Blend

1.9 ounces/54 g
    lavender 40/42
1.0 ounce/28 g
    peppermint
    2nd distilled

Colorant

1 tablespoon/15 mL
    madder root dispersed
    into 3 tablespoons/
    45 mL olive oil

Additive

6.6 ounces/187 g
    buttermilk

Safe Soaping!

Wear proper safety gear the whole time · Work in a well-ventilated space · No distractions

Use Any Milk

As with all these recipes, you can substitute any other kind of milk or dairy product,
used in the same amount.

Make the Soap Batter

1 Measure the olive oil into a glass bowl large enough to hold the full recipe with room to mix. Heat the oil to 105°F (40.5°C) and set aside.

2 Measure the distilled water and the lye into separate heatproof containers. Add the lye to the water a tablespoon (15 mL) at a time (never add the liquid to the lye). Stir continuously until the lye fully dissolves and the water becomes clear. Stir the sodium lactate into the lye-water.

3 When the oil and the lye-water have cooled to about 105°F (40.5°C), add the lye-water to the oils, pouring it over the shaft of the stick blender to minimize air bubbles.

4 Insert the stick blender into the batter, tilting it so that any trapped air can escape. *Do not turn on the stick blender until the blades are fully immersed.* Alternate pulsing and stirring with the stick blender until a very thin trace is achieved.

5 Add the buttermilk and essential oil blend. Stir in with a whisk.

Color and Pour

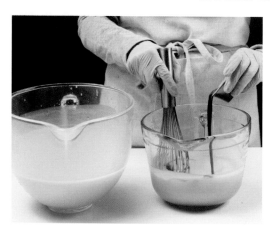 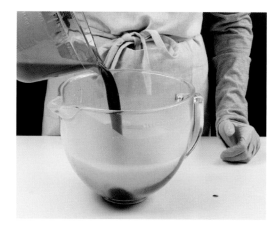

6 Pour 20 ounces (567 g) of uncolored batter into the second bowl and add the madder root. Mix well with a whisk.

7 Pour the colored batter back into the first bowl. Pour from several inches above the bowl, using a circular motion so that the two batters swirl together.

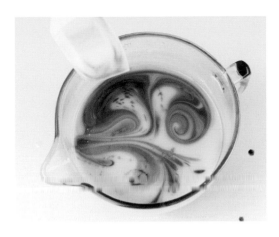

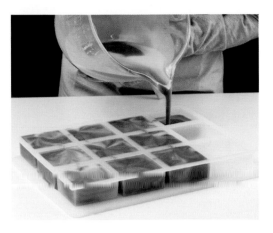

8 Stir the swirled batter one time with a spatula. Do not overmix the swirl.

9 Fill the mold by pouring into a corner of each cavity. Pour into the same spot until the entire cavity is full; do not move the bowl around as you pour.

Final Steps

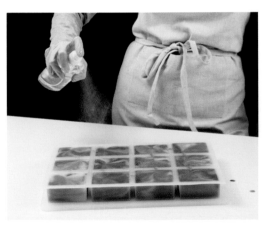

Spray thoroughly with 99% rubbing alcohol several times over 90 minutes to prevent soda ash. Let the soap sit at room temperature for at least 48 hours before unmolding. Once the soaps are unmolded, let them sit another 24 hours before beveling the top four edges of the bars.

Let the bars cure in a well-ventilated area for at least 6 weeks before using, turning them every few days to ensure they cure evenly. **Note:** The madder root will lighten as the soap cures.

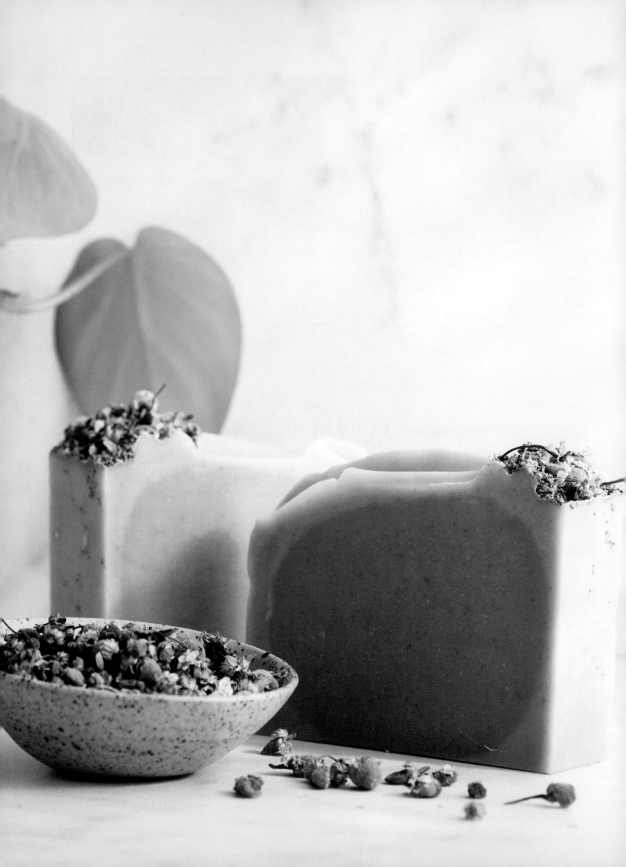

Textured Turmeric Bars
with Banana Milk

50% ADDED AT TRACE • MAKES 8 BARS

The addition of banana milk (a slurry of banana and water) and turmeric gives this soap a slightly exfoliating texture. Since the milk is not strained, the natural color variation is part of the unique design. The natural sugar from the fruit contributes to a creamy and stable lather, but it also means that the soap gets quite hot in the making. To combat this, keep your temperatures low and put the soap in the freezer after pouring to avoid partial gel. This recipe traces quickly, which helps achieve the textured tops.

Mold and Special Tools
10-inch (25 cm) silicone
loaf mold
Spoon for texturing top

Oil Amounts
8.5 ounces/241 g
pure olive oil (25%)
7.8 ounces/221 g
coconut oil (23%)
6.8 ounces/193 g
sunflower seed oil (20%)
5.8 ounces/164 g
babassu oil (17%)

1.7 ounces/48 g
avocado butter (5%)
1.7 ounces/48 g
shea butter (5%)
1.7 ounces/48 g
castor oil (5%)

Lye-Water
5.6 ounces/159 g
distilled water
4.9 ounces/139 g
lye (4% superfat)
3 teaspoons/15 mL
sodium lactate

Essential/Oil
2.5 ounces/71 g
orange 10×

Colorant
2 teaspoons/10 mL
turmeric powder

Additives
5.6 ounces/159 g
banana milk
1–2 tablespoons/15–30 mL
chamomile buds

Prepare Ahead

Make the banana milk by blending 1 medium banana (about 1 cup mashed) with 3 cups (710 mL) distilled water until very smooth. This milk does not need to be strained.

Safe Soaping!

Wear proper safety gear the whole time · Work in a well-ventilated space · No distractions

Use Any Milk

As with all these recipes, you can substitute any other kind of milk or dairy product, used in the same amount.

Make the Soap Batter

1 Melt the babassu oil in its original container and measure it into a heatproof bowl large enough to hold the entire recipe. Melt and measure the coconut oil and add it to the bowl. Add the avocado butter and shea butter to the hot oils and stir until melted. If needed, microwave the bowl in 10-second bursts to melt the butter completely. Add the olive oil, sunflower seed oil, and castor oil and set the bowl aside.

2 Measure the distilled water and the lye into separate heatproof containers. Add the lye to the water a tablespoon (15 mL) at a time (never add the liquid to the lye). Stir continuously until the lye fully dissolves and the water becomes clear. Stir the sodium lactate into the lye-water.

3 When the oils and the lye-water have cooled to about 105°F (40.5°C), add the lye-water to the oils, pouring it over the shaft of the stick blender to minimize air bubbles.

4 Insert the stick blender into the batter, tilting it so that any trapped air can escape. *Do not turn on the stick blender until the blades are fully immersed.* Stick-blend until you reach emulsion.

Mix and Pour

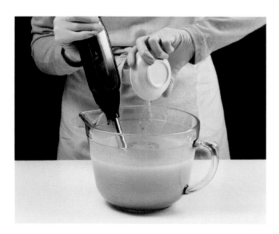

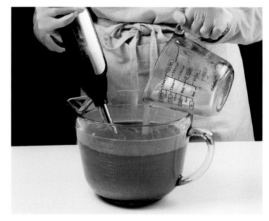

5 Add the turmeric powder, trapping it under the stick blender head as you insert the blender into the batter so it doesn't puff up out of the bowl when you turn the blades on. Blend until incorporated and the batter is at thin trace.

6 Add the orange essential oil and banana milk. Stick-blend until incorporated. The banana milk will cause the batter to thicken quickly.

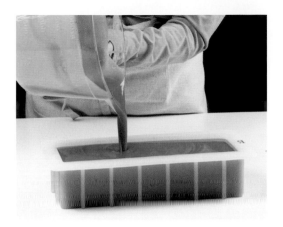

7 Pour or spoon the batter into the mold.

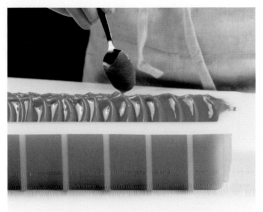

8 Texture the top by using the back of a spoon to push batter from one side of the mold to the other. Make one long side of the soap taller than the other.

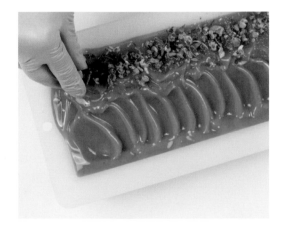

9 Sprinkle the chamomile along the taller side of the loaf. Press very slightly with a gloved finger, just enough to ensure it stays in the batter.

Final Steps

Spray thoroughly with 99% rubbing alcohol several times over 90 minutes to prevent soda ash. Place the mold in the freezer overnight to prevent partial gel. Remove from the freezer and unmold. Let the loaf sit another 48 hours before slicing. Frozen soaps tend to soften quite a bit as they thaw and need time to harden again.

To cut the loaf, put it on its side, with the chamomile against the cutting surface. You want the herbs to be the last thing the blade passes through, otherwise they will be pulled through the loaf and leave drag marks.

Let the bars cure in a well-ventilated area for 4 to 6 weeks before using, turning them every few days to ensure they cure evenly.

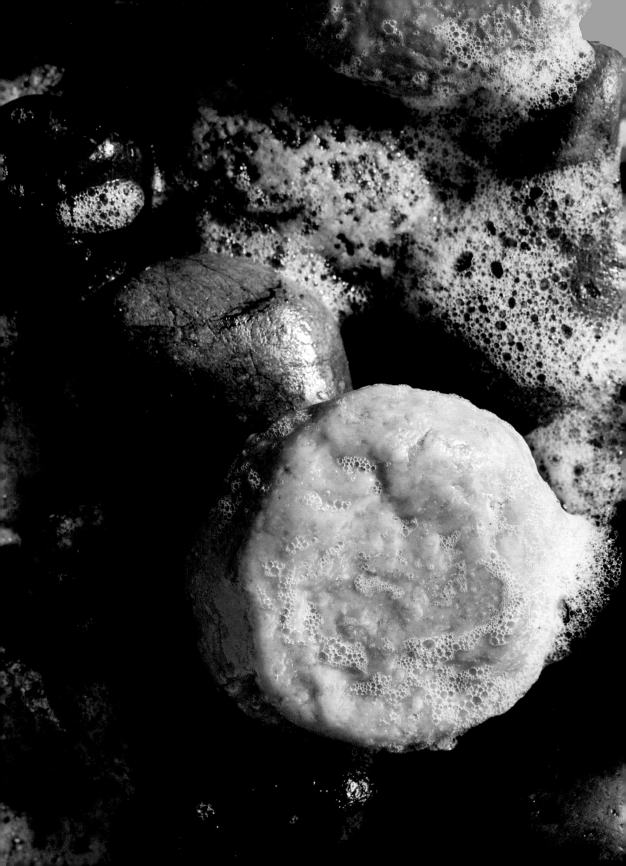

Hand-Sculpted Soap Stones
with Split Pea Milk

50% ADDED AT TRACE • MAKES 5 BARS

This unique design uses a softer recipe so that you can hand-sculpt intriguing soap "stones." Split pea milk, a supersustainable vegan milk high in DHA omega-3 fatty acids, is the latest "milk du jour." This soap takes a little longer to cure than most, but it eventually hardens into wonderful soaps.

Molds and Special Tools

4 mini round silicone column molds
4 easy-pour containers
Rubber bands

Oil Amounts

3.2 ounces/91 g sweet almond oil (20%)
3.2 ounces/91 g rice bran oil (20%)
2.4 ounces/68 g coconut oil (15%)
1.6 ounces/45 g babassu oil (10%)
1.6 ounces/45 g canola oil (10%)
0.9 ounce/26 g mango butter (6%)
0.8 ounce/23 g chia seed oil (5%)
0.8 ounce/23 g jojoba oil (5%)
0.8 ounce/23 g macadamia nut oil (5%)
0.6 ounce/17 g castor oil (4%)

Lye-Water

2.6 ounces/74 g distilled water
2.1 ounces/60 g lye (4% superfat)
1 teaspoon/5 mL sodium lactate

Essential Oil Blend

0.8 ounce/23 g grapefruit
0.3 ounce/8.5 g patchouli

Colorants

Disperse each into 1 tablespoon/15 mL distilled water.

1 teaspoon/5 mL purple Brazilian clay
1 teaspoon/5 mL natural Brazilian clay
1 teaspoon/5 mL pink Brazilian clay
1 teaspoon/5 mL yellow silt clay

Additive

2.6 ounces/74 g split pea milk

Safe Soaping!

Wear proper safety gear the whole time · Work in a well-ventilated space · No distractions

Use Any Milk

As with all these recipes, you can substitute any other kind of milk or dairy product, used in the same amount.

Prepare Ahead

Assemble the molds by pressing along the edges to ensure the seals are closed tightly and there are no gaps. Group them together with rubber bands and stand them upright in an extra container, as shown in step 8.

Split Pea Milk

1 cup (237 mL) dried split peas

12 cups (2,839 mL) distilled water

1. Combine the peas and 4 cups (946 mL) of the water in a medium saucepan and bring to a boil. Boil for 10 minutes. Reduce the heat and simmer until tender, about 1 hour.

2. Combine the cooked peas and the cooking water with the remaining 8 cups (1,893 mL) water in a blender and blend until completely smooth.

3. Store in the refrigerator for up to 4 days or freeze for longer storage. Stir before using as milk; it will separate.

Make the Soap Batter

1 Melt the babassu oil in its original container and measure it into a heatproof bowl large enough to hold the entire recipe. Melt and measure the coconut oil and add it to the bowl. Add the mango butter to the hot oils and stir until melted. If needed, microwave the bowl in 10-second bursts to melt the butter completely. Add the canola oil, chia seed oil, jojoba oil, macadamia nut oil, rice bran oil, sweet almond oil, and castor oil and set the bowl aside.

2 Measure the distilled water and the lye into separate heatproof containers. Add the lye to the water a tablespoon (15 mL) at a time (never add the liquid to the lye). Stir continuously until the lye fully dissolves and the water becomes clear. Stir the sodium lactate into the lye-water.

3 When the oils and the lye-water have cooled to about 105°F (40.5°C), add the lye-water to the oils, pouring it over the shaft of the stick blender to minimize air bubbles.

4 Insert the stick blender into the batter, tilting it so that any trapped air can escape. *Do not turn on the stick blender until the blades are fully immersed.* Alternate pulsing and stirring with the stick blender until you reach emulsion.

5 Add the split pea milk and the essential oil blend. Stick-blend until combined, keeping trace thin.

Color and Pour

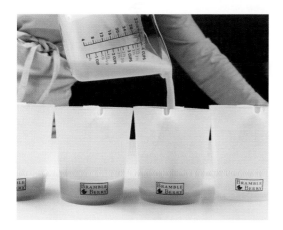

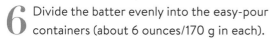

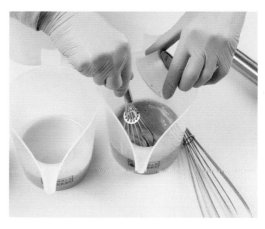

6 Divide the batter evenly into the easy-pour containers (about 6 ounces/170 g in each).

7 Add one clay to one of the containers and mix well with a whisk.

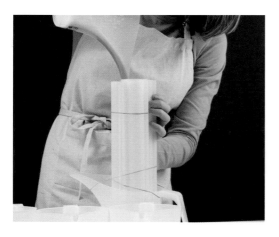

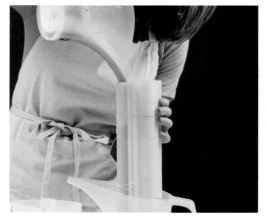

8 Pour the colored batter into one of the column molds.

9 Repeat with the other three clays, pouring each one as soon as the color is mixed in. Let sit in the molds at room temperature for 24 hours.

Sculpt the Soap

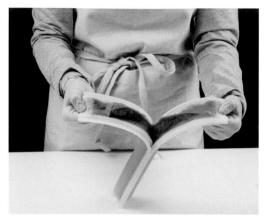

10 Wearing gloves, unmold the soaps — they will still be very soft.

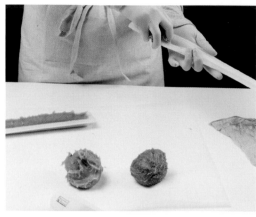

11 Scoop the batter from each mold and roll it into a rough ball.

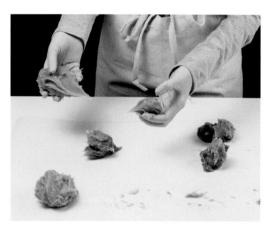

12 Divide each ball into five equal pieces, sticking the pieces together to create five multicolored blobs.

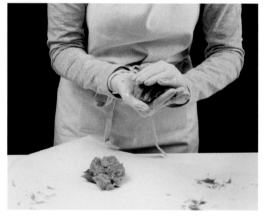

13 Mold each blob into a round "stone." Spray your gloved hands and/or the soaps liberally with 99% rubbing alcohol as you sculpt to prevent the batter from sticking to the gloves, making for smoother stones and less muddied colors. If needed, change gloves, or wash and dry your gloved hands between each stone.

Final Steps

Set the soaps on parchment paper to cure in a well-ventilated area for 8 to 10 weeks. Turn them every few days to ensure they harden evenly.

Faux Funnel Pour
with Camel's Milk

100% REPLACEMENT • MAKES 8 BARS

This beautiful, easy-to-make recipe uses a round column mold to create an interesting pattern of concentric circles. Camel's milk is associated with skin softening; its alpha hydroxy acids and vitamin C have antiaging and anti-inflammation properties. In soap, the milk produces a rich, stable lather.

Mold and Special Tools
Silicone column mold
3 easy-pour containers
Fine-mesh strainer

Oil Amounts
9.1 ounces/258 g
 coconut oil (35%)
5.2 ounces/147 g
 apricot kernel oil (20%)
3.9 ounces/111 g
 sunflower seed oil (15%)
3.9 ounces/111 g
 macadamia nut oil (15%)
2.6 ounces/74 g
 mango butter (10%)
1.3 ounces/37 g
 castor oil (5%)

Lye Mixture
8.5 ounces/241 g
 camel's milk, frozen
3.6 ounces/102 g
 lye (6% superfat)
2 teaspoons/10 mL
 sodium lactate

Fragrance Oil
1.9 ounces/54 g
 Shave and a Haircut

Essential Oil Alternative
1.9 ounces/54 g lime

Colorants
Disperse each into 1 table-spoon/15 mL sunflower seed oil.

1 teaspoon/5 mL
 ultraviolet blue pigment
1 teaspoon/5 mL
 hydrated chrome
 green oxide

Safe Soaping!
Wear proper safety gear the whole time · Work in a well-ventilated space · No distractions

Use Any Milk
As with all these recipes, you can substitute any other kind of milk or dairy product, used in the same amount.

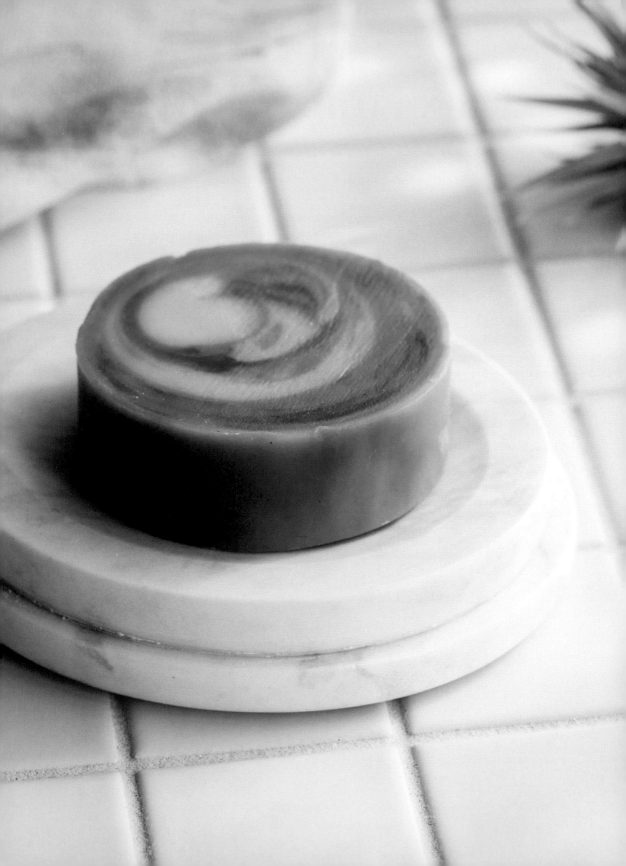

Prepare Ahead

Assemble the silicone mold, pressing along the edges to seal them tightly.

Make the Soap Batter

1 Melt and measure the coconut oil into a heatproof bowl large enough to hold the entire recipe. Add the mango butter to the hot coconut oil and stir until melted. If needed, microwave the bowl in 10-second bursts until the mango butter is melted. Add the apricot kernel oil, macadamia nut oil, sunflower seed oil, and castor oil and set the bowl aside.

2 Measure the frozen milk and the lye into separate heatproof containers. Slowly add the lye to the milk a tablespoon (15 mL) at a time, stirring continuously until all the lye has fully dissolved. This can take up to 30 minutes due to the cold temperature. Add the sodium lactate to the lye mixture and stir to combine.

3 When the oils have cooled to between 100 and 105°F (38–40.5°C) and the lye mixture is between 75 and 85°F (24–29°C), gently pour the lye mixture through the strainer into the oils, stirring any residue gently with a spatula.

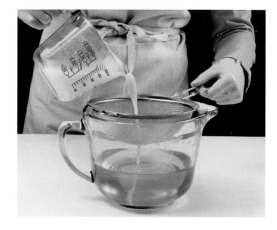

4 Insert the stick blender into the batter, tilting it so that any trapped air can escape. *Do not turn on the stick blender until the blades are fully immersed.* Alternate pulsing and stirring with the stick blender until a thin trace is achieved.

5 Add the fragrance oil to the batter and stir by hand to combine.

Color and Pour

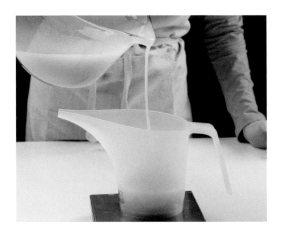

6 Divide the batter evenly among three easy-pour containers, about 12 ounces (340 g) in each.

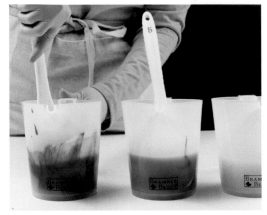

7 Add 1 teaspoon (5 mL) of dispersed ultraviolet blue to one container and 1 teaspoon (5 mL) of dispersed hydrated chrome green oxide to a second container; leave the third container plain.

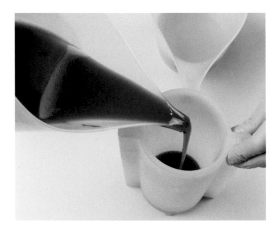

8 Pour about an inch (2.5 cm) of the blue soap batter into the center of the mold.

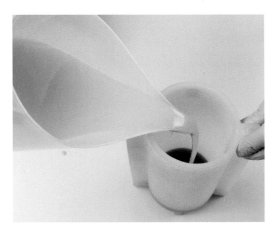

9 Pour about an inch (2.5 cm) of white batter into the center of the mold.

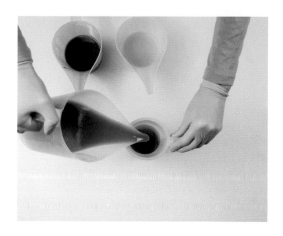

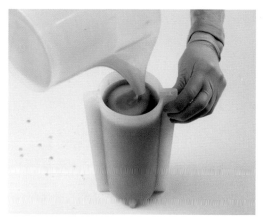

10 Pour about an inch (2.5 cm) of green batter into the center of the mold.

11 Keep pouring into the center of the mold, alternating the three colors until it's full.

Final Steps

Let the soap sit at room temperature for 48 hours before unmolding. Slice into bars with a knife.

Let the bars cure in a well-ventilated area for 4 to 6 weeks before using, turning them every few days so that they cure evenly.

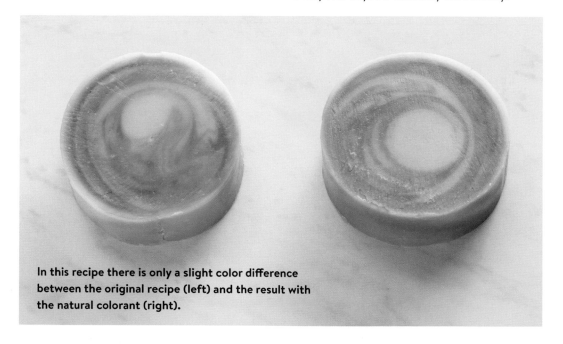

In this recipe there is only a slight color difference between the original recipe (left) and the result with the natural colorant (right).

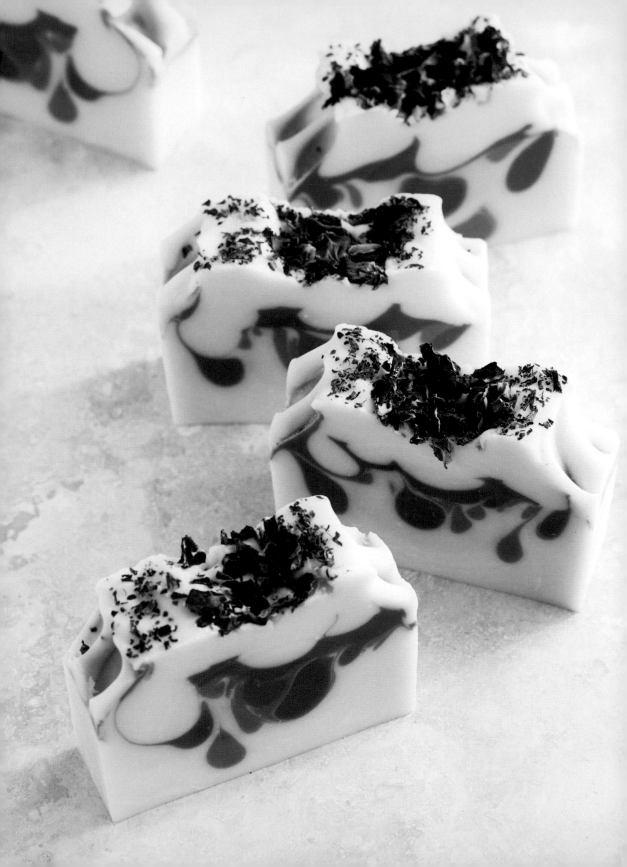

Drop Swirls
with Kefir and Rose Petals

30% added at trace • Makes 8 bars

This beautiful batch utilizes a stunning drop swirl to achieve its design, which is enhanced with a sprinkle of rose petals. Kefir gives the recipe all the natural goodness of milk with an added probiotic boost. These bars go in the freezer overnight to prevent overheating.

Mold and Special Tools

10-inch (25.4 cm) silicone loaf mold
3 easy-pour containers
Small spoon for texturing tops

Oil Amounts

6.8 ounces/193 g
 coconut oil (20%)
6.8 ounces/193 g
 canola oil (20%)
6.8 ounces/193 g
 rice bran oil (20%)
5.1 ounces/145 g
 babassu oil (15%)
3.4 ounces/96 g
 macadamia nut oil (10%)
1.7 ounces/48 g
 borage oil (5%)
1.7 ounces/48 g
 kokum butter (5%)
1.7 ounces/48 g
 castor oil (5%)

Lye-Water

7.9 ounces/224 g
 distilled water
4.6 ounces/113 g
 lye (7% superfat)
3 teaspoons/15 mL
 sodium lactate

Fragrance Oil

2.4 ounces/68 g
 Pomegranate and
 Black Currant

Essential Oil Alternative
1.9 ounces/54 g
 Valencia orange
0.5 ounce/14 g
 Egyptian geranium

Colorant

Disperse each into 1 table-spoon/15 mL canola oil.

1 teaspoon/5 mL
 titanium dioxide

1 teaspoon/5 mL
 bronze mica
1 teaspoon/5 mL
 raspberry mica

Natural Colorant Alternative
¼ teaspoon/1.2 mL
 brown oxide
2 teaspoons/9.9 mL
 ultramarine pink pigment

Additives

3.3 ounces/94 g
 kefir
3 tablespoon/45 mL
 dried rose petals
1 tablespoon/15 mL
 finely ground dried rose petals (or use dust from the bottom of the bag)

Safe Soaping!

Wear proper safety gear the whole time · Work in a well-ventilated space · No distractions

Use Any Milk

As with all these recipes, you can substitute any other kind of milk or dairy product, used in the same amount.

Prepare Ahead

Make the kefir. If you use commercial kefir, choose an unflavored one with as few additives as possible.

Make the Soap Batter

1 Melt the babassu oil in its original container and measure it into a heatproof bowl large enough to hold the entire recipe. Melt and measure the coconut oil and add it to the bowl. Add the kokum butter to the hot oils and stir until melted. If needed, microwave the bowl in 10-second bursts to melt the butter completely. Add the borage oil, canola oil, macadamia nut oil, rice bran oil, and castor oil and set the bowl aside.

2 Measure the distilled water and the lye into separate heatproof containers. Add the lye to the water a tablespoon (15 mL) at a time (never add the liquid to the lye). Stir continuously until the lye fully dissolves and the water becomes clear. Stir the sodium lactate into the lye-water.

3 When the oils and the lye-water have cooled to about 105°F (40.5°C), add the lye-water to the oils, pouring it over the shaft of the stick blender to minimize air bubbles.

4 Insert the stick blender into the batter, tilting it so that any trapped air can escape. *Do not turn on the stick blender until the blades are fully immersed.* Alternate pulsing and stirring with the stick blender until the mix is lightly emulsified.

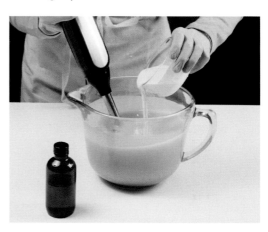

5 Add the kefir and fragrance oil. Stick-blend to thin trace.

Color the Soap

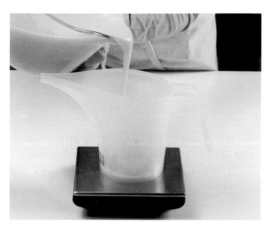

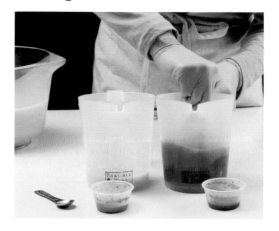

6 Pour 8 ounces (227 g) soap batter into one easy-pour container and 4 ounces (113 g) into a second easy-pour container.

7 Stir in 1 teaspoon (5 mL) raspberry mica into the larger amount of batter.

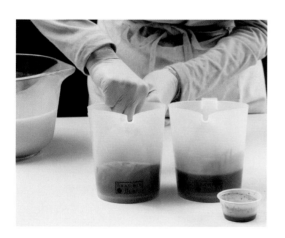

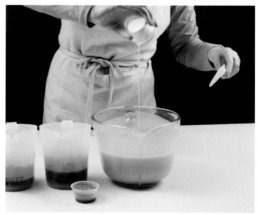

8 Stir in ½ teaspoon (2.5 mL) bronze mica into the smaller amount.

9 Add all of the dispersed titanium dioxide to the remaining batter and stir well.

Pour the Soap

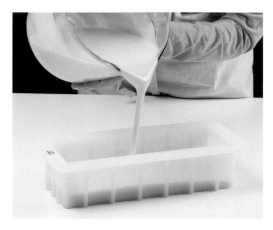

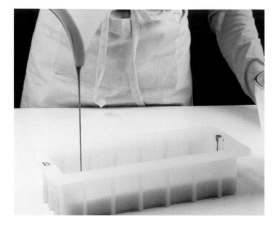

10 Pour the white batter into the mold until it is about half full. Transfer the remaining white batter into an easy-pour container.

11 Pour all of the bronze soap batter into the white batter, making lines down the length of the mold. Hold the container high enough so that the color breaks through the white layer.

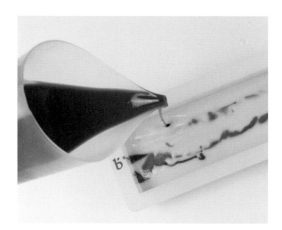

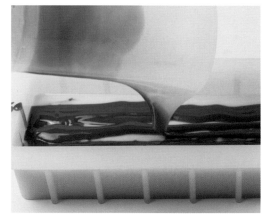

12 Pour two-thirds of the raspberry batter on top of the bronze, again making lines down the length of the mold. Hold the container slightly closer this time, but still high enough to break through.

13 Pour the remaining raspberry batter even closer to the mold, so that it layers instead of breaking through.

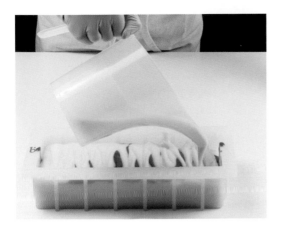

14 Pour the remaining white batter on top, breaking through just slightly with your lines. Cover the loaf so that all you see is white batter.

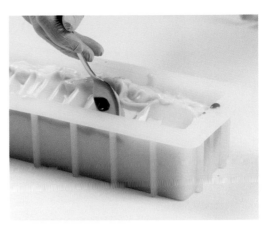

15 Texture the top by dragging a small spoon along the outer edges of the soap, then up and into the center. If it is too thin to texture, let it sit for a couple of minutes. (Depending on how deep you texture, you may pull up some pink batter on the sides as well.)

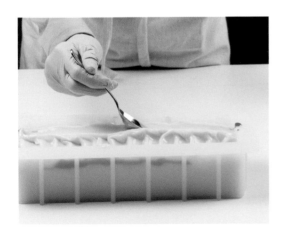

16 Smooth the spoon down the center of the mold to create a wide, slightly flattened line.

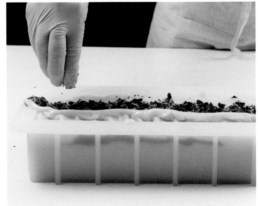

17 Sprinkle the 3 tablespoons (45 mL) of rose petals down the center of the loaf. Use 1 tablespoon (15 mL) of crushed rose petals to fill in around the textured edges and to fill any gaps in the center. Press the petals in gently with your finger so they don't fall off when unmolding and slicing.

Final Steps

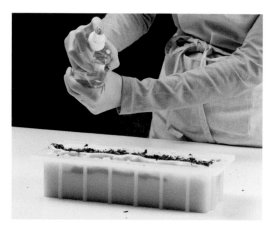

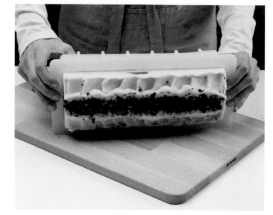

18 Spray thoroughly with 99% rubbing alcohol to prevent soda ash. Put the mold in the freezer overnight to prevent overheating. Remove from the freezer and let harden for 48 hours before unmolding. Frozen soaps tend to soften quite a bit as they thaw and need time to harden again.

19 Slice these bars on their sides or upside down to prevent the rose petals from leaving drag lines through the bars.

20 Let the bars cure in a well-ventilated area for 4 to 6 weeks before using, turning them every few days to ensure they cure evenly.

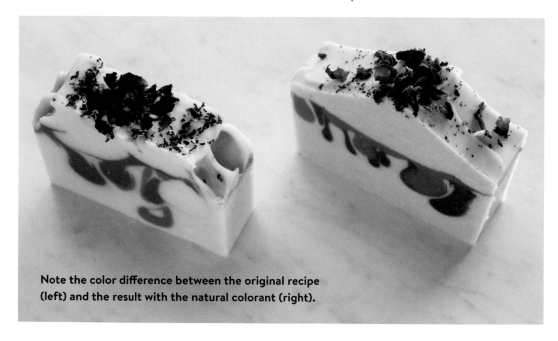

Note the color difference between the original recipe (left) and the result with the natural colorant (right).

Cupcake Soaps
with Whipped Cream

30% ADDED AT TRACE • MAKES 6 CUPCAKES

These soaps aren't just good looking — they're packed with skin-loving cocoa butter. They also contain a whopping 30 percent homemade whipped cream to give these bars a smooth, conditioning feel when used. (Commercial whipped cream has added sugar, which you don't want here.) Specially cut fondant mats create a wrapperlike design for the base of the cupcakes, and jojoba beads are sprinkled on top for decoration.

Mold and Special Tools
Round silicone cupcake mold
Textured silicone fondant mat
Template for cupcake
   wrappers (6)
1M frosting tip
Disposable frosting bag
Easy-pour or other container
   for propping the frosting
   bag while filling

Oil Amounts
10.5 ounces/283 g
   palm oil (30%)
10.5 ounces/283 g
   coconut oil (30%)
5.2 ounces/147 g
   cocoa butter (15%)
3.5 ounces/99 g
   kokum butter (10%)

1.7 ounces/48 g
   palm kernel flakes (5%)
1.7 ounces/48 g
   olive pomace oil (5%)
1.7 ounces/48 g
   castor oil (5%)

Lye-Water
8.1 ounces/230 g
   distilled water
4.9 ounces/139 g
   lye (7% superfat)
3 teaspoons/15 mL
   sodium lactate

Fragrance Oils
Do not blend these.

1.1 ounces/31 g
   Vanilla Select
1.4 ounces/40 g
   Pure Honey

Essential Oil Alternative
1.5 ounces/43 g
   lemon
0.2 ounce/5.7 g
   cinnamon

Colorant
1 teaspoon/5 mL brown
   oxide dispersed into
   1 tablespoon/15 mL
   olive pomace oil

Additives
3.4 ounces/96 g
   whipped cream
¼ teaspoon/1.25 mL
   jasmine jojoba beads

Safe Soaping!
Wear proper safety gear the whole time · Work in a well-ventilated space · No distractions

Use Any Milk
As with all these recipes, you can substitute any other kind of milk or dairy product, used in the same amount.

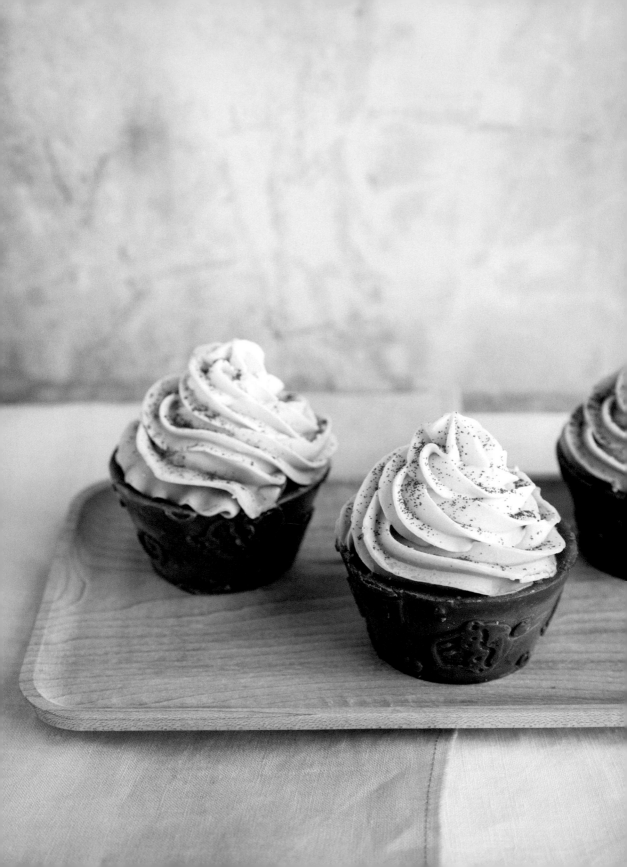

Prepare Ahead

Cut the tip off of the frosting bag and insert the frosting tip.

Line the Mold

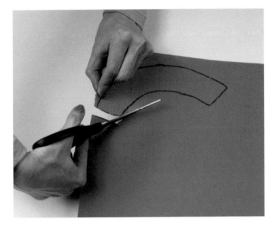

1 Use the template to trace and cut out six cupcake wrappers from the fondant mat.

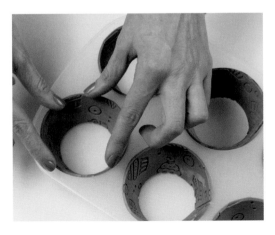

2 Line each cavity in the cupcake mold with a wrapper, patterns facing in.

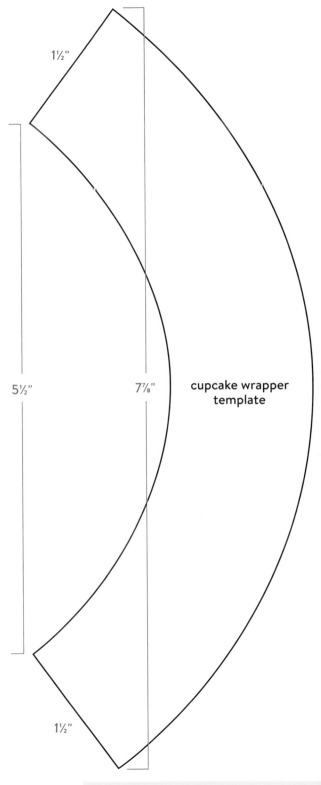

1½"

5½"   7⅞"

cupcake wrapper template

1½"

Make the Soap Batter

1 Melt the palm oil in its original container, mix it thoroughly, and measure it into a heatproof bowl large enough to hold the entire recipe. Melt and measure the coconut oil and add it to the bowl. Add the cocoa butter, kokum butter, and palm kernel flakes to the hot oils and stir until melted. If needed, microwave the bowl in 10-second bursts to melt the butter completely. Add the olive pomace oil and castor oil and set the bowl aside. Measure out the whipped cream and leave at room temperature until ready to use.

2 Measure the distilled water and the lye into separate heatproof containers. Add the lye to the water a tablespoon (15 mL) at a time (never add the liquid to the lye). Stir continuously until the lye fully dissolves and the water becomes clear. Stir the sodium lactate into the lye-water.

3 When the oils and the lye-water have cooled to about 105°F (40.5°C), add the lye-water to the oils, pouring it over the shaft of the stick blender to minimize air bubbles.

4 Insert the stick blender into the batter, tilting it so that any trapped air can escape. *Do not turn on the stick blender until the blades are fully immersed.* Alternate pulsing and stirring with the stick blender until a thin trace is achieved.

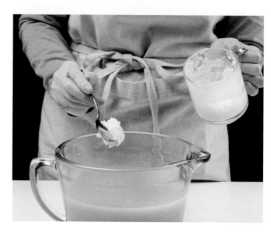

5 Add the whipped cream to your soap batter and whisk in until fully incorporated.

Color and Pour

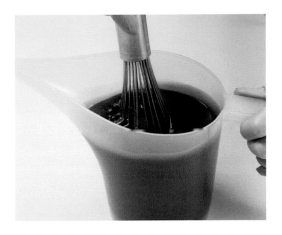

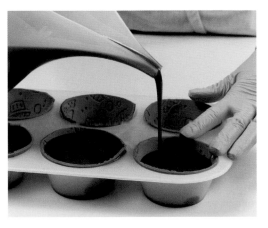

6 Pour 22 ounces (624 g) of batter into a separate container, then add the Vanilla Select fragrance oil and ½ teaspoon (2.5 mL) of dispersed brown oxide; stir well with a whisk.

7 Pour the brown batter into the mold, filling the cavities to the top of the liners.

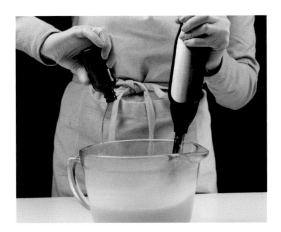

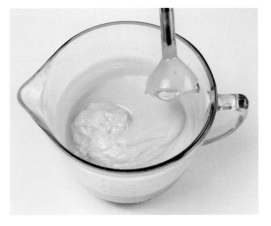

8 Add the Pure Honey fragrance oil to the remaining uncolored batter and stick-blend until you achieve a thick trace; you want thick, pipeable batter to "frost" the cupcakes.

9 Let the batter continue to thicken, checking on it every couple minutes. Giving the white batter a few minutes to thicken also gives the brown batter time to set in the mold and better support the weight of the frosting.

Pipe the Soap

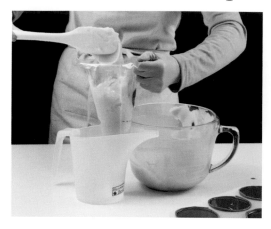

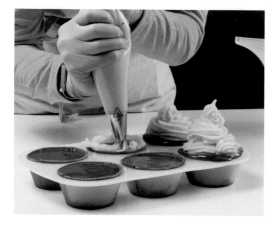

10 Once the batter is thick enough to hold its shape without melting back down, use a spatula to scoop it into the frosting bag.

11 Pipe a generous amount of frosting onto each cupcake, moving in a circle to build up a peak. This recipe makes plenty of frosting, so feel free to pipe tall peaks.

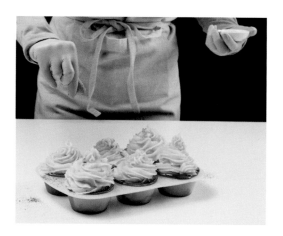

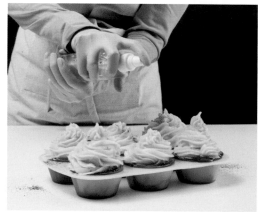

12 Sprinkle the tops of the cupcakes with the jojoba beads.

13 Spray thoroughly with 99% rubbing alcohol several times over 90 minutes to prevent soda ash. Let the soaps sit for at least 48 hours at room temperature before unmolding.

Final Steps

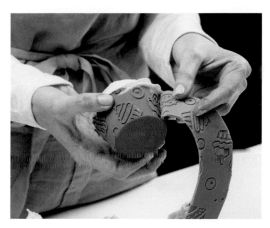

14 Unmold the cupcakes and gently peel back the liners. If the liners do not peel away smoothly, let them sit unmolded for another 24 hours, then try again.

15 Let the soaps cure in a well-ventilated area for 4 to 6 weeks before using, turning them every few days to ensure they cure evenly.

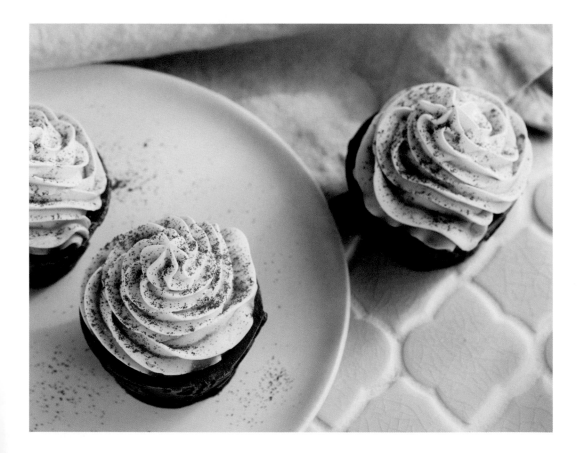

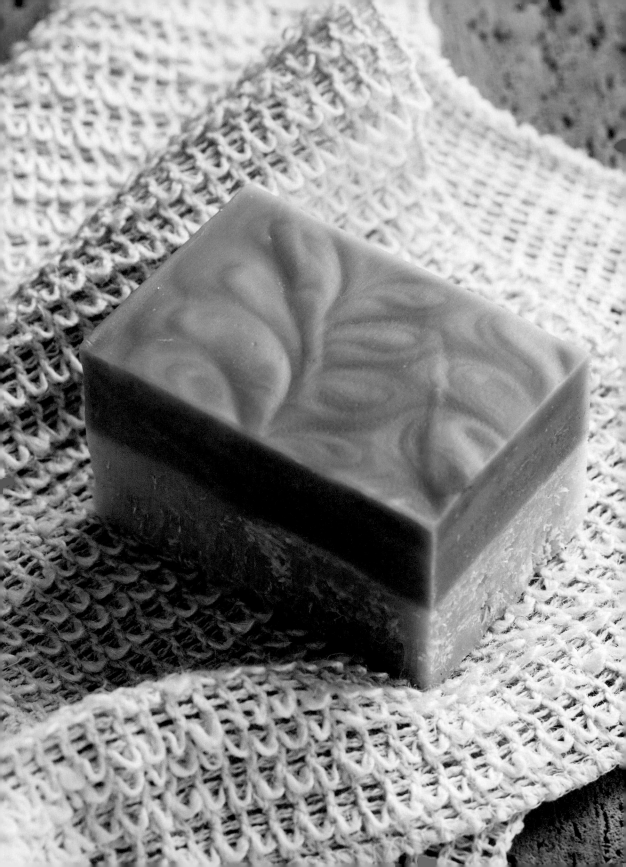

Loofah and Swirls
with Sheep's Milk

50% ADDED AT TRACE • MAKES 6 BARS

This two-layer soap is made with luxurious sheep's milk. It's a dual-purpose bar, with an exfoliating layer on one side and a smooth side for when you don't want as much scrubbing. It is made in a flat, horizontal mold that creates bars that fit perfectly in your hand.

Mold and Special Tools
6-inch (15 cm) silicone slab mold
3 easy-pour containers
Chopstick

Oil Amounts
5.4 ounces/153 g coconut oil (20%)
5.4 ounces/153 g sweet almond oil (20%)
4.0 ounces/113 g babassu oil (15%)
4.0 ounces/113 g canola oil (15%)
2.7 ounces/76 g meadowfoam oil (10%)
1.9 ounces/54 g kukui nut oil (7%)
1.3 ounces/37 g kokum butter (5%)
1.3 ounces/37 g shea butter (5%)
0.8 ounce/23 g castor oil (3%)

Lye-Water
4.5 ounces/128 g distilled water
3.7 ounces/105 g lye (7% superfat)
2½ teaspoons/12.5 mL sodium lactate

Fragrance Oil
1.9 ounces/54 g Sparkling Snowdrop

Essential Oil Alternative
0.9 ounce/26 g lavender 40/42
1 ounce/28 g lemon

Colorants
Disperse each into 1 tablespoon/15 mL sweet almond oil

1 teaspoon/5 mL Blue Slushy mica
1 teaspoon/5 mL Lavender mica

Natural Colorant Alternative
1 teaspoon/5 mL ultramarine blue pigment
1 teaspoon/5 mL ultramarine violet pigment

Additives
4.4 ounces/125 g sheep's milk
2 tablespoons (28 grams) shredded loofah

Safe Soaping!
Wear proper safety gear the whole time · Work in a well-ventilated space · No distractions

Use Any Milk
As with all these recipes, you can substitute any other kind of milk or dairy product, used in the same amount.

Make the Soap Batter

1 Melt the babassu oil in its original container and measure it into a heatproof bowl large enough to hold the entire recipe. Melt and measure the coconut oil and add it to the bowl. Add the kokum butter and shea butter to the hot oils and stir until melted. If needed, microwave the bowl in 10-second bursts to melt the butter completely. Add the canola oil, kukui nut oil, meadowfoam oil, sweet almond oil, and castor oil and set the bowl aside.

2 Measure the distilled water and the lye into separate heatproof containers. Add the lye to the water a tablespoon (15 mL) at a time (never add the liquid to the lye). Stir continuously until the lye fully dissolves and the water becomes clear. Stir the sodium lactate into the lye-water.

3 When the oils and the lye-water have cooled to about 105°F (40.5°C), add the lye-water to the oils, pouring it over the shaft of the stick blender to minimize air bubbles.

4 Insert the stick blender into the batter, tilting it so that any trapped air can escape. *Do not turn on the stick blender until the blades are fully immersed.* Alternate pulsing and stirring with the stick blender until a very thin trace is achieved.

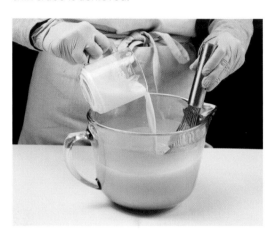

5 Add the sheep's milk to the batter and whisk until incorporated.

Color and Swirl

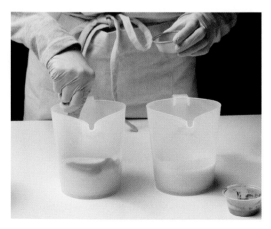

6 Pour the batter into three easy-pour containers and color as follows, stirring each by hand:
- Container 1: 19 ounces (539 g) batter with the shredded loofah
- Container 2: 10 ounces (283 g) batter with 1 teaspoon (5 mL) Blue Slushy mica
- Container 3: 10 ounces (283 g) batter with 1 teaspoon (5 mL) Lavender mica

Note: The Sparkling Snowdrop fragrance oil causes mild acceleration. Be ready to pour and swirl quickly.

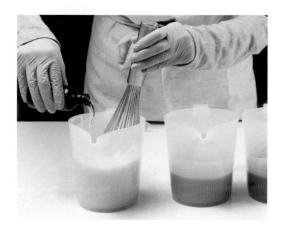

7 Add about half of the Sparkling Snowdrop fragrance oil to the batter with the shredded loofah. Mix well with a whisk.

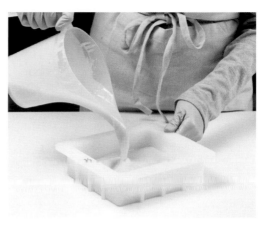

8 Pour all of the white batter into the mold.

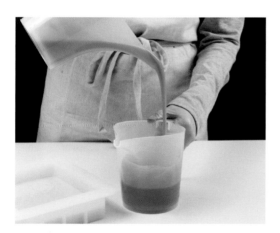

9 Divide the rest of the fragrance oil equally between the blue and purple batters and mix well. Pour the blue batter into the purple batter, holding the blue container at different heights and pouring in a circular motion to swirl the batters together. Reserve a couple spoonfuls of the blue batter for swirling the top of the loaf.

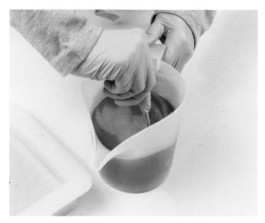

10 Give the swirled batter a single stir with a spoon. Don't overmix the swirl.

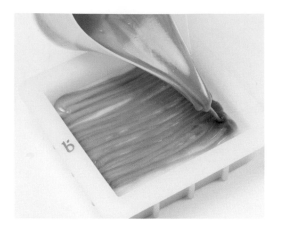

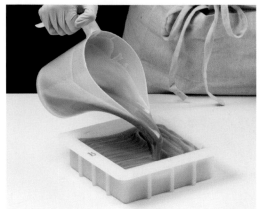

11 Pour the swirled batter onto the white batter, pouring low and slow so you don't break through. Tap the mold on the counter to flatten the top layer.

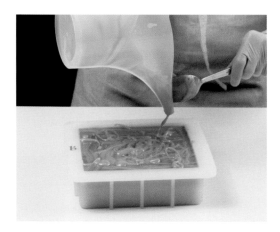

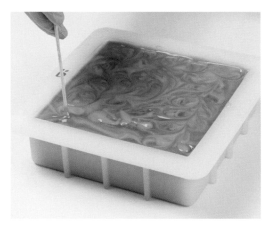

12 Use your reserved blue batter to make swirls of batter along the top of the loaf.

13 Create small infinity symbols on the surface using the chopstick.

Final Steps

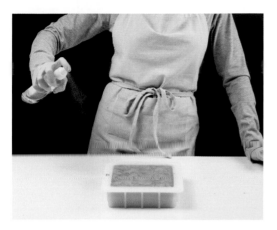

14 Spray thoroughly with 99% rubbing alcohol several times over 90 minutes to prevent soda ash. Let the soap sit at room temperature and wait 48 hours before unmolding and slicing.

15 Use a large knife to slice the loaf in half, then slice each half into three bars.

16 Let the bars cure in a well-ventilated area for 4 to 6 weeks before using, turning the bars every few days to ensure they cure evenly.

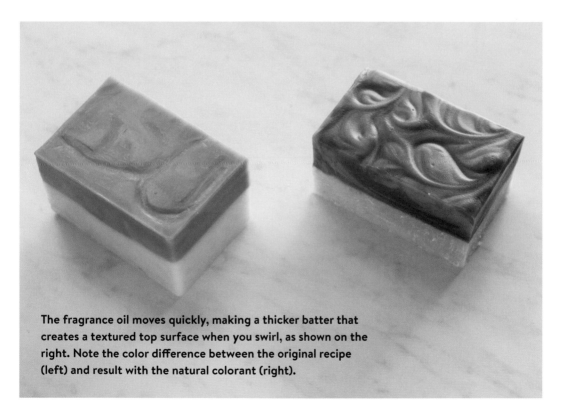

The fragrance oil moves quickly, making a thicker batter that creates a textured top surface when you swirl, as shown on the right. Note the color difference between the original recipe (left) and result with the natural colorant (right).

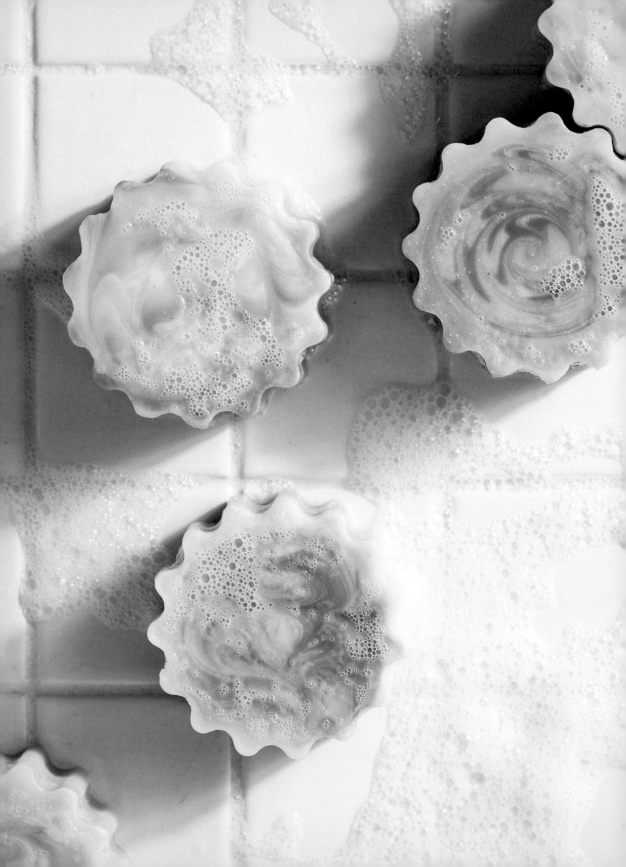

Dead Sea-Salt
Brine Bar

Salt hardens soap bars. Dead Sea salt can be obtained only from the Dead Sea in Jordan and Israel. Because it is loaded with skin-enhancing minerals, it can cause weeping when added straight to soap batter. For this recipe, we dissolve the salt in the lye-water to give all the benefits of a salt bar without adding any scratchiness.

This is an all-natural bar with a refreshing spearmint-eucalyptus scent. Salt naturally inhibits lather, so this recipe has a high coconut percentage (90%) and high superfat (20%) to compensate for the extra cleansing and oil-stripping abilities of the coconut oil. This recipe is also unusual in that it uses a higher percentage of water than normal to fully dissolve both the lye and the salt. This recipe can move fast, so be prepared!

Mold and Special Tools
Round scalloped silicone mold
Fine-mesh strainer
2 easy-pour containers
Chopstick

Oil Amounts
14.4 ounces/408 g
    coconut oil (90%)
0.8 ounce/23 g
    canola oil (5%)
0.8 ounce/23 g
    castor oil (5%)

Lye-Water
3.2 ounces/91 g
    distilled water
2.2 ounces/62 g
    lye (20% superfat)
0.6 ounce/17 g
    Dead Sea salt

Essential Oil Blend
0.7 ounce/20 g
    spearmint
0.4 ounce/11 g
    eucalyptus

Colorant Amounts
Disperse each into 1 table-spoon/15 mL canola oil.

1 teaspoon/5 mL
    green chrome oxide
1 teaspoon/5 mL
    titanium dioxide

Additive
2.6 ounces/74 g
    raw milk

Safe Soaping!
Wear proper safety gear the whole time · Work in a well-ventilated space · No distractions

Use Any Milk
As with all these recipes, you can substitute any other kind of milk or dairy product, used in the same amount.

Make the Soap Batter

1 Melt and measure the coconut oil into a heatproof bowl large enough to hold the entire recipe. Add the canola oil and castor oil and set the bowl aside.

2 Measure the distilled water and the lye in separate heat-resistant containers. Add the lye to the water a tablespoon (15 mL) at a time (never add the liquid to the lye). Stir continuously as the lye dissolves and the water becomes clear.

3 As soon as all the lye is dissolved, add the Dead Sea salt to the lye-water and stir to dissolve. This may take a while, as the water will be very saturated.

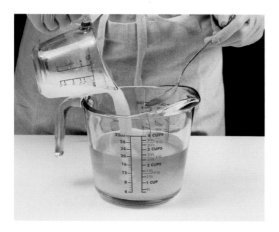

4 Once the oils and lye mixture have cooled to 105°F (40°C; rewarm the oils in the microwave if needed) and the salt has fully dissolved, gently pour the lye-water into the oils. Insert the stick blender into the batter, tilting the shaft to release any air that might be caught under the blades.

Do not turn on the stick blender until the blades are fully immersed. Alternate pulsing and stirring with the stick blender until a very thin trace is achieved.

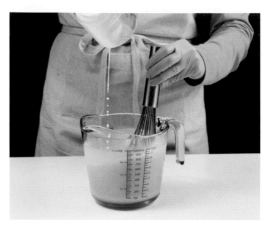

5 Add the raw milk and essential oil blend and whisk to combine.

Color and Swirl

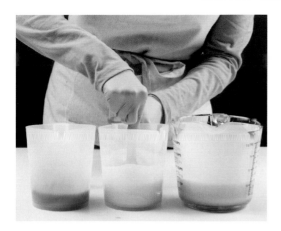

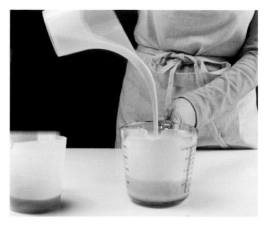

6 Pour the following amounts of batter and colorant into the easy-pour containers and whisk to combine:
- 8 ounces (227 g) soap batter plus 1 teaspoon (5 mL) dispersed titanium dioxide
- 4 ounces (113 g) soap batter plus ¼ teaspoon dispersed green chrome oxide

7 Pour the white batter back into the bowl of plain batter. Pour from varying heights in a circular pattern so that they swirl together.

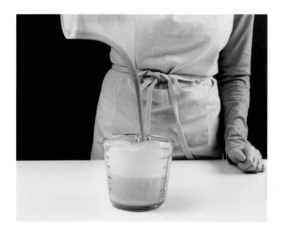

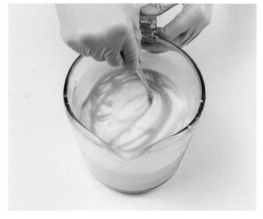

8 Repeat with the green batter.

9 Stir the batter once with a spoon. Do not overmix the swirl.

Pour the Soap

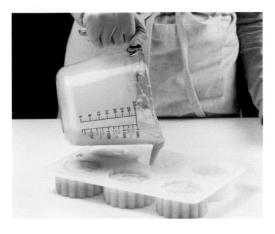

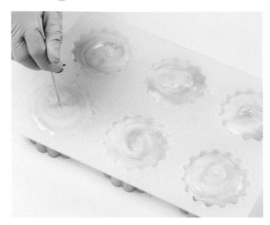

10 Pour the batter into the mold, dividing it evenly among the cavities.

11 In a single spiral motion, swirl the top of each cavity with a chopstick.

Final Steps

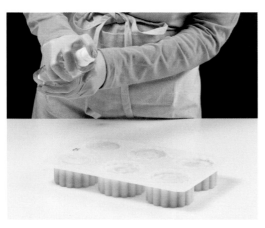

Spray thoroughly with 99% rubbing alcohol several times over 90 minutes to prevent soda ash. Let set for at least 8 hours at room temperature before unmolding. If unmolding is difficult, try again in an hour or two. (Salt bars harden quickly and can usually be unmolded the same day.)

Let the bars cure in a well-ventilated area for 4 to 6 weeks before using, turning them every few days to ensure they cure evenly.

Poppy Seeds
and Swirls

100% REPLACEMENT • MAKES 8 BARS

With a generous serving of mango and shea butter to provide skin conditioning, this is a dual-texture and -color soap. The striking design uses a divider to produce even lines. You can make your own divider with clear packing tape and cardboard or use soap-safe premade ones.

Mold and Special Tools
10-inch (25 cm) silicone loaf mold with dividers
Fine-mesh strainer
2 easy-pour containers
Soap beveller (optional)

Oil Amounts
8.2 ounces/232 g coconut oil (25%)
8.2 ounces/232 g palm oil (25%)
6.6 ounces/187 g sunflower seed oil (20%)
3.3 ounces/94 g apricot kernel oil (10%)
3.3 ounces/94 g mango butter (10%)
1.6 ounces/45 g shea butter (5%)
1.6 ounces/45 g castor oil (5%)

Lye Mixture
10.9 ounces/309 g milk, frozen
4.6 ounces/130 g lye (5% superfat)
3 teaspoons/15 mL sodium lactate

Fragrance Oil
2.4 ounces/68 g Bergamot Black Tea

Essential Oil Alternative
2 ounces/57 g patchouli

Colorant
1 teaspoon/5 mL black oxide dispersed into 1 tablespoon/15 mL sunflower seed oil

Additive
1½ teaspoons/7.5 mL poppy seeds

Prepare Ahead

Insert the two end dividers in the mold and then the center divider. Make sure they are pressed tight against the bottom of the mold.

Safe Soaping!
Wear proper safety gear the whole time · Work in a well-ventilated space · No distractions

Use Any Milk
As with all these recipes, you can substitute any other kind of milk or dairy product, used in the same amount.

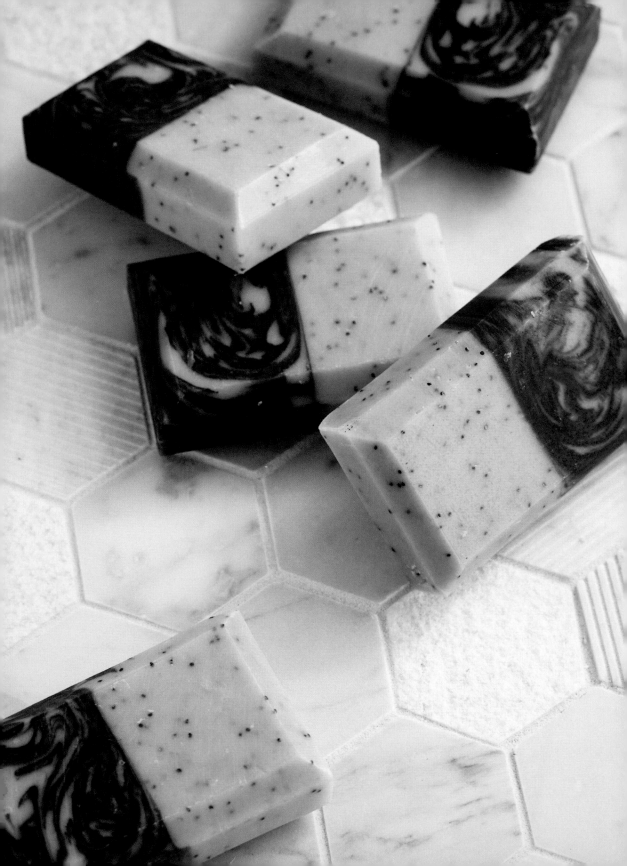

Make the Soap Batter

1 Melt the palm oil in its original container, mix it thoroughly, and measure it into a heatproof bowl large enough to hold the entire recipe. Melt and measure the coconut oil and add it to the bowl. Add the shea butter and mango butter to the hot oils and stir until melted. If needed, microwave the bowl in 10-second bursts to melt the butter completely. Add the apricot kernel oil, castor oil, and sunflower seed oil and set the bowl aside.

2 Measure the frozen milk and the lye into separate heatproof containers. Slowly add the lye to the milk a tablespoon (15 mL) at a time, stirring continuously until all the lye has fully dissolved. This can take up to 30 minutes due to the cold temperature.

Add the sodium lactate to the lye mixture and stir to combine.

3 When the oils have cooled to between 100 and 105°F (38–40.5°C) and the lye mixture is between 75 and 85°F (24–29°C), gently pour the lye mixture through the strainer into the oils, stirring any residue gently with a spatula.

4 Insert the stick blender into the batter, tilting it so that any trapped air can escape. *Do not turn on the stick blender until the blades are fully immersed.* Alternate pulsing and stirring with the stick blender until a thin trace is achieved.

5 Stir in the fragrance oil.

Color and Pour

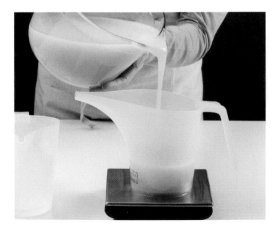

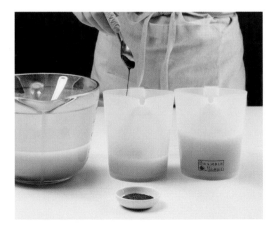

6 Pour 17 ounces (482 g) soap batter into an easy-pour container.

7 Pour 7.5 ounces (213 g) soap batter into another easy-pour container and add ½ teaspoon (5 mL) dispersed black oxide.

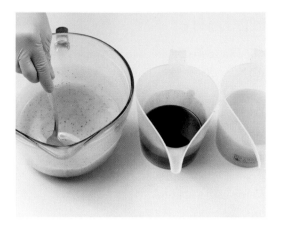

8 Stir the poppy seeds into the remaining batter.

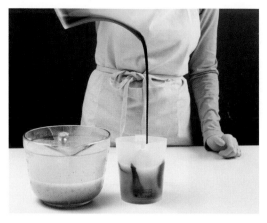

9 Pour the black batter into the white batter in a circular motion, holding the container up so the black batter sinks in. Stir the batter once. Do not overmix.

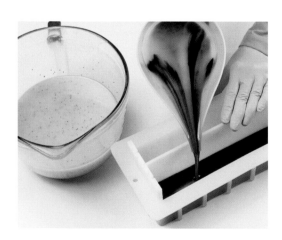

10 Pour the black-and-white-swirled soap into one half of the mold.

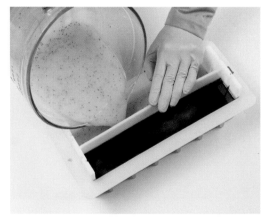

11 Pour the poppy-seed batter into the other half.

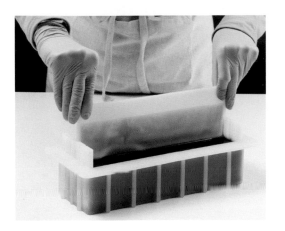
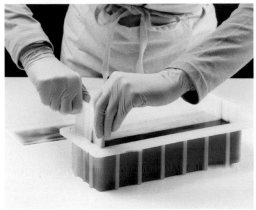

12 Carefully lift the dividers straight up and out of the mold. Leave the tops as they are — do not swirl the black-and-white batters.

Final Steps

Spray thoroughly with 99% rubbing alcohol several times over 90 minutes to prevent soda ash. Let sit at room temperature for 48 hours before unmolding.

Unmold, slice into bars, and bevel the edges, if desired.

Let the bars cure in a well-ventilated area for 4 to 6 weeks before using, turning them every few days to ensure they cure evenly. **Note:** The bars will turn light tan as they cure.

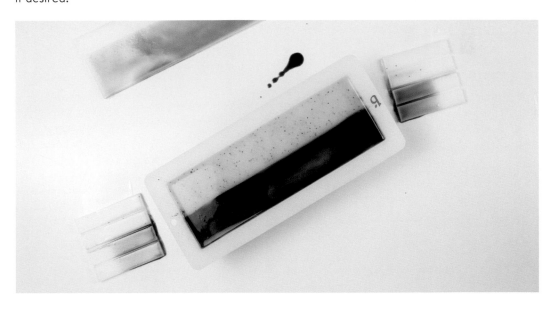

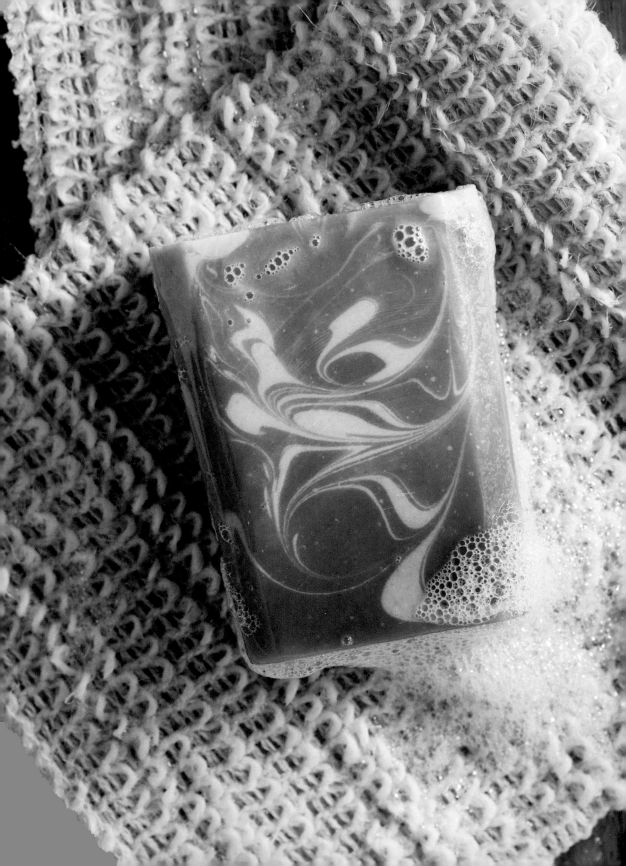

Hangered Drop Swirls
with Colloidal Oatmeal and Honey

100% REPLACEMENT • MAKES 10 BARS

This bar uses a classic beauty blend of oats, milk, and honey. The whole milk nourishes skin while the honey enhances lather and the oats soothe and protect gentle skin. Colloidal oatmeal is so finely ground that it feels smooth in the final bar, with no scrubbiness. This recipe is considered a "bastille" bar, which means it's a traditional castile bar (with lots of olive oil) plus a touch of coconut oil and castor oil to help with lather. It does need extra cure and hardening time thanks to the large amount of olive oil in the recipe.

The swirls are created by drop-swirl and hand-swirl techniques. The swirl design will pop out more as the fragranced parts darken.

Mold and Special Tools

Tall 12-inch (30.5 cm)
  silicone loaf mold
Fine-mesh strainer
2 easy-pour containers
Hanger swirl tool
  (see page 130)
Chopstick
Soap beveller (optional)

Oil Amounts

27.2 ounces/771 g
  pure olive oil (80%)
5.1 ounces/145 g
  coconut oil (15%)
1.7 ounces/48 g
  castor oil (5%)

Lye Mixture

11.2 ounces/318 g
  whole milk, frozen
4.4 ounces/125 g
  lye (7% superfat)
3 teaspoons/15 mL
  sodium lactate

Fragrance Oil

1.8 ounces/51 g
  Oatmeal, Milk, and Honey

Essential Oil Alternative
1.2 ounces/34 g
  Valencia orange
0.6 ounce/17 g
  frankincense

Colorants

Disperse both into 1 tablespoon/15 mL olive oil.

1 teaspoon/5 mL
  titanium dioxide
1 teaspoon/5 mL
  Sunset Orange mica

Natural Colorant Alternative
Replace the orange mica with 1 teaspoon/5 mL of a dispersed blend of 1 part yellow oxide to 2 parts ultramarine pink pigment.

Additives

2.4 ounces/68 g
  colloidal oatmeal
3 teaspoons/15 m honey

Safe Soaping!

Wear proper safety gear the whole time · Work in a well-ventilated space · No distractions

Use Any Milk

As with all these recipes, you can substitute any other kind of milk or dairy product, used in the same amount.

Make the Soap Batter

1 Melt and measure the coconut oil into a heatproof bowl large enough to hold the entire recipe. Add the olive oil and castor oil and set the bowl aside.

2 Measure the frozen milk and the lye into separate heatproof containers. Slowly add the lye to the milk a tablespoon (15 mL) at a time, stirring continuously until all the lye has fully dissolved. This can take up to 30 minutes due to the cold temperature. Add the sodium lactate to the lye mixture and stir to combine.

3 When the oils have cooled to between 100 and 105°F (38–40.5°C) and the lye mixture is between 75 and 85°F (24–29°C), gently pour the lye mixture through the strainer into the oils, stirring any residue gently with a spatula.

4 Insert the stick blender into the batter, tilting it so that any trapped air can escape. *Do not turn on the stick blender until the blades are fully immersed.* Alternate pulsing and stirring with the stick blender until you reach emulsion.

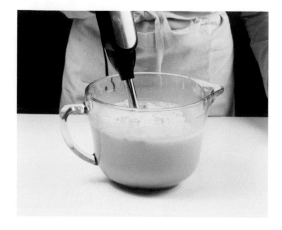

5 Add the honey and colloidal oatmeal and pulse with the stick blender until both are fully incorporated and the batter is at thin trace.

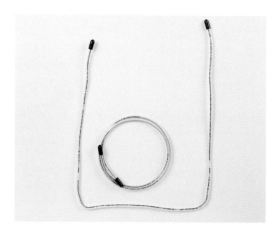

You can buy a flexible swirling tool like this or fashion one from a wire hanger that you bend to fit your mold.

Color and Pour

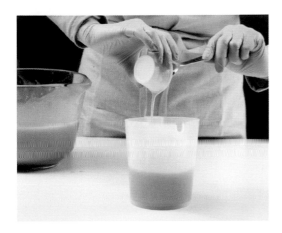

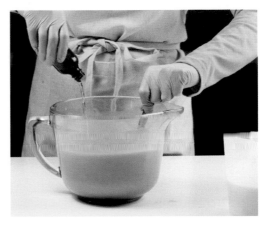

6 Pour 12 ounces (340 g) of batter into an easy-pour container and add all of the dispersed titanium dioxide. Stir in well and set aside.

7 Add the fragrance oil to the remaining batter and stir well by hand.

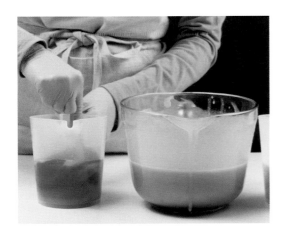

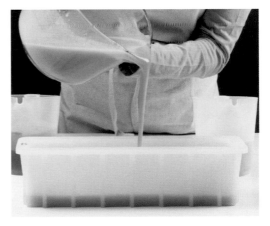

8 Pour 7 ounces (198 g) of the fragranced batter into a second easy-pour container and add 1 teaspoon (5 mL) dispersed Sunset Orange mica. Stir well.

9 Pour one-third of the remaining uncolored batter into the mold.

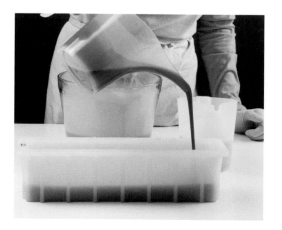
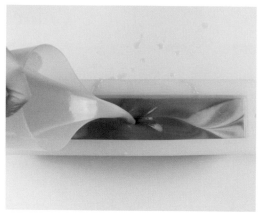

10 Make drop swirls in the mold by alternately pouring the orange and white batters, using about one-third of each. Pour lines down the length of the mold, pouring from higher up so that the layers break through.

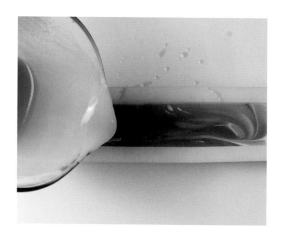
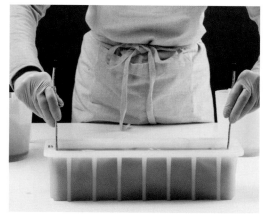

11 Pour lines of uncolored batter over the orange and white lines. Repeat the whole cycle two more times. Reserve a few ounces (about 100 g) of uncolored batter for the final layer and a couple spoonfuls of orange and white batter for the top design.

12 Insert the hanger swirl tool along the side of the mold and push it to the bottom.

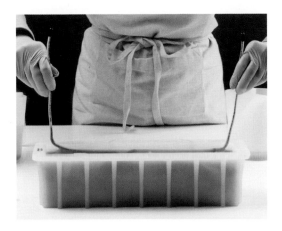

13 Moving the tool away from the side of the mold, make three or four large, overlapping circles without breaking the surface of the batter.

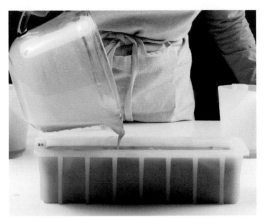

14 Cover the entire mold with the rest of the uncolored batter, pouring low and slow to avoid breaking through or disturbing the swirls.

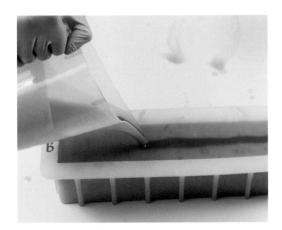

15 To make the top design, pour one thin line of orange batter down the center of the loaf.

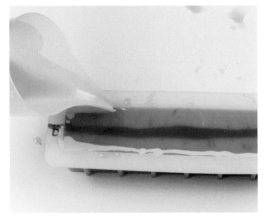

16 Pour a thin line of white batter down each side of the loaf. (There should be uncolored batter showing between the orange and white lines.)

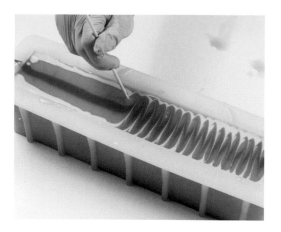

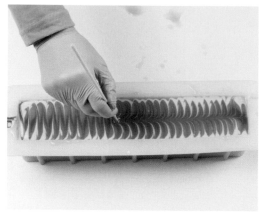

17 Insert a chopstick slightly into the top layer and swirl it from side to side of the mold.

18 Use the chopstick to pull a line down the center of the swirl. Remove it from the mold, then pull a line along each long side of the mold.

Final Steps

Spray thoroughly with 99% rubbing alcohol several times over 90 minutes to prevent soda ash. Let sit at room temperature for at least 48 hours before unmolding. Slice into bars and bevel the longer edges of the soaps, if desired.

Let the bars cure in a well-ventilated area for 6 to 8 weeks before using, turning them every few days to ensure they cure evenly.

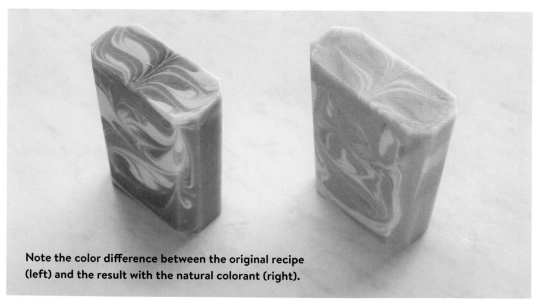

Note the color difference between the original recipe (left) and the result with the natural colorant (right).

Layered Coffee
and Cream Bars

30% ADDED AT TRACE • MAKES 6 BARS

Instead of water, this soap uses cooled coffee, which is high in antioxidants and adds a smoky base note to the soap. In addition, we've amped up the recipe with coffee oil. Because cream is especially high in fat, we add it at trace. This fun design is created with a mold made from two-part silicone putty, readily available online and in craft stores. We first saw a coffee bean design on Mila Breeze's (of Jasminka Soaps) Instagram page and were inspired to make our own version.

If you prefer a completely natural version, go fragrance-free and enjoy the soft scent of the natural coffee ingredients. Skip the gold mica dusting.

Mold and Special Tools

Two-part molding putty
Vinyl gloves (latex gloves will stick to the putty)
Freezer paper
2 ounces/57 g
    whole coffee beans
2-pound (907 g) wood loaf mold with silicone liner
Powder duster
3 easy-pour containers

Oil Amounts

5.5 ounces/156 g
    coconut oil (25%)
5.5 ounces/156 g
    palm oil (25%)
5.5 ounces/156 g
    canola oil (25%)

2.2 ounces/62 g
    coffee butter (10%)
1.1 ounces/31 g
    coffee oil (5%)
1.1 ounces/31 g
    palm kernel flakes (5%)
1.1 ounces/31 g castor oil (5%)

Lye Mixture

4.5 ounces/128 g
    chilled coffee
3.1 ounces/88 g
    lye (4% superfat)
2 teaspoons/10 mL
    sodium lactate

Fragrance Oil

1.6 ounces/45 g
    Espresso

Colorants

1 teaspoon/5 mL titanium dioxide dispersed into 1 tablespoon/15 mL canola oil
1 teaspoon/5 mL
    brown oxide dispersed into 1 tablespoon/15 mL canola oil
2 teaspoons/10 mL
    Gold Sparkle mica, not dispersed (for dusting)

Additive

2.0 ounces/57 g
    cream
1 teaspoon/5 mL brewed coffee grounds

Safe Soaping!

Wear proper safety gear the whole time · Work in a well-ventilated space · No distractions

Use Any Milk

As with all these recipes, you can substitute any other kind of milk or dairy product, used in the same amount.

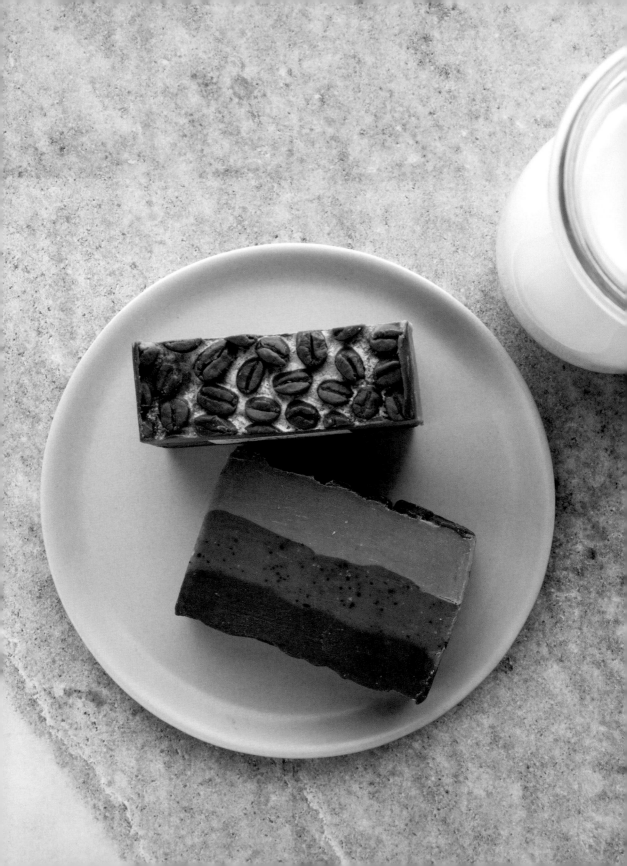

Make the Liner

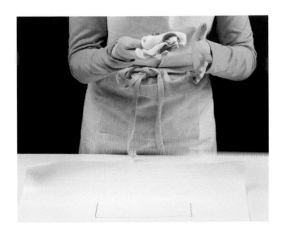

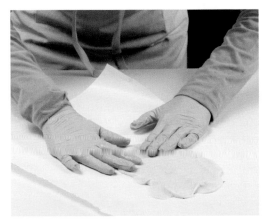

1 Trace the outline of the mold onto a piece of freezer paper. Following the directions, mold the two containers of putty until well combined.

2 Flatten the putty onto the freezer paper until it covers the outline of the mold (you will trim it to fit).

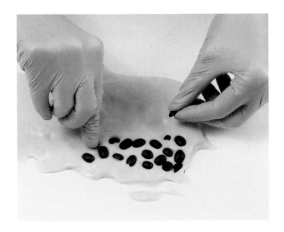

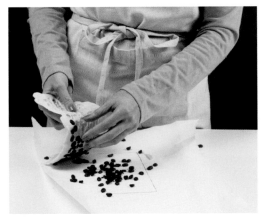

3 Working quickly, push the coffee beans, seam-side down, into the putty. Push the beans in far enough to get a good impression without breaking through the layer of putty. Cover the entire surface.

4 Let dry for 1 to 2 hours, then peel off the freezer paper and remove the beans. Wash the liner to remove any bean particles. Trim with scissors to fit into the mold. Insert the liner smooth-side down into the mold, then insert the regular liner into the wooden mold.

Make the Soap Batter

1 Melt the palm oil in its original container, mix it thoroughly, and measure it into a heatproof bowl large enough to hold the entire recipe. Melt and measure the coconut oil and add it to the bowl. Add the palm kernel flakes and coffee butter to the hot oils and stir until melted. If needed, microwave the bowl in 10-second bursts to melt the butter completely. Add the coffee oil, castor oil, and canola oil and set the bowl aside. Measure the cream into a small container and set it aside.

2 Measure the coffee and the lye into separate heatproof containers. Add the lye to the coffee a tablespoon (15 mL) at a time (never add the liquid to the lye). Stir continuously until the lye fully dissolves. Stir the sodium lactate into the lye solution.

3 When the oils and the lye solution have cooled to about 105°F (40.5°C), add the lye solution to the oils, pouring it over the shaft of the stick blender to minimize air bubbles.

4 Insert the stick blender into the batter, tilting it so that any trapped air can escape. *Do not turn on the stick blender until the blades are fully immersed.* Alternate pulsing and stirring with the stick blender until a thin trace is achieved.

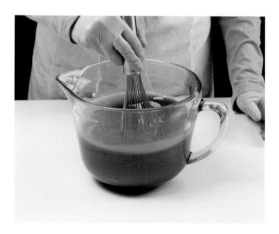

5 Add the cream and the fragrance oil and mix in with a whisk.

Color and Pour

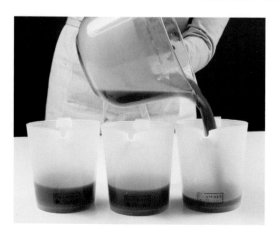

6 Divide the batter equally into three easy-pour containers (put about 10 ounces/283 g in each container).

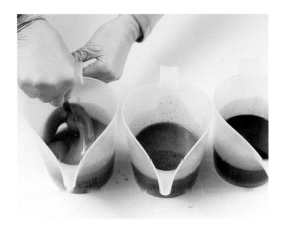

7 Add ½ teaspoon (2.5 mL) of the dispersed brown oxide to one container, the teaspoon (5 mL) of coffee grounds to the second, and 1 teaspoon (5 mL) of the dispersed titanium dioxide to the third. Stick-blend each container for just a few seconds to speed up trace. This recipe will thicken quickly on its own, so don't overdo it.

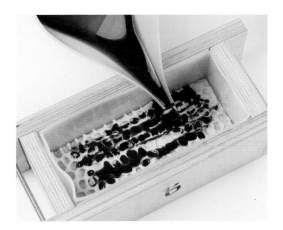

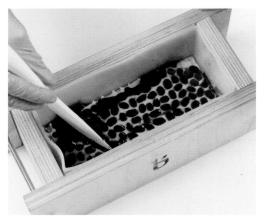

8 Pour a little of the dark brown batter into the mold, just enough to fill in the indentations. Scrape the batter in a couple different directions with a spatula and tap the mold to fill each crevice. Scrape excess batter out of the mold.

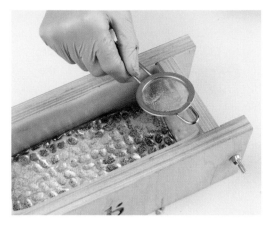

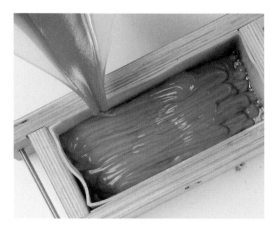

9 Place the Gold Sparkle mica into the powder duster and gently tap it over the soap to lightly dust the surface of the liner and the coffee beans. If the mica layer is too thick, the beans will not adhere to the soap.

10 Pour the entire container of the lightest batter into the mold, pouring low and slow to make a smooth layer. Tap the mold on the counter to flatten the soap.

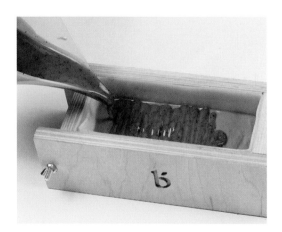

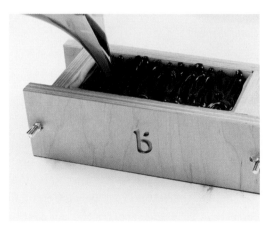

11 Pour the batter with the coffee grounds, again pouring low and slow to create a second layer without breaking through the first. Tap the mold on the counter to flatten the soap.

12 Pour a third layer with the darkest batter, again pouring low and slow without breaking through. Tap the mold on the counter to flatten the soap.

TECHNIQUE TIP

It can help to pour each layer slowly over the back of a spatula to keep the layers from breaking through.

Final Steps

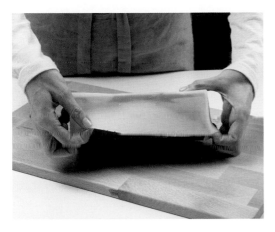

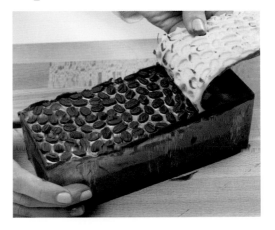

13 Spray thoroughly with 99% rubbing alcohol several times over 90 minutes to prevent soda ash. Let sit at room temperature for 48 hours before unmolding.

14 Unmold the soap and gently peel away the liner. If it won't peel away easily, wait another 24 hours.

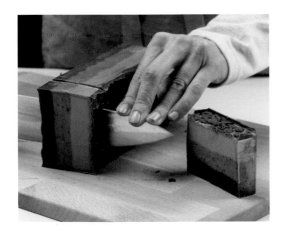

15 Place the loaf on its side before slicing into bars. This prevents the coffee grounds from leaving drag lines when you cut the soap.

16 Let the bars cure in a well-ventilated area for 4 to 6 weeks before using, turning them every few days to ensure they cure evenly. **Note:** These bars will darken as they cure due to the fragrance oil.

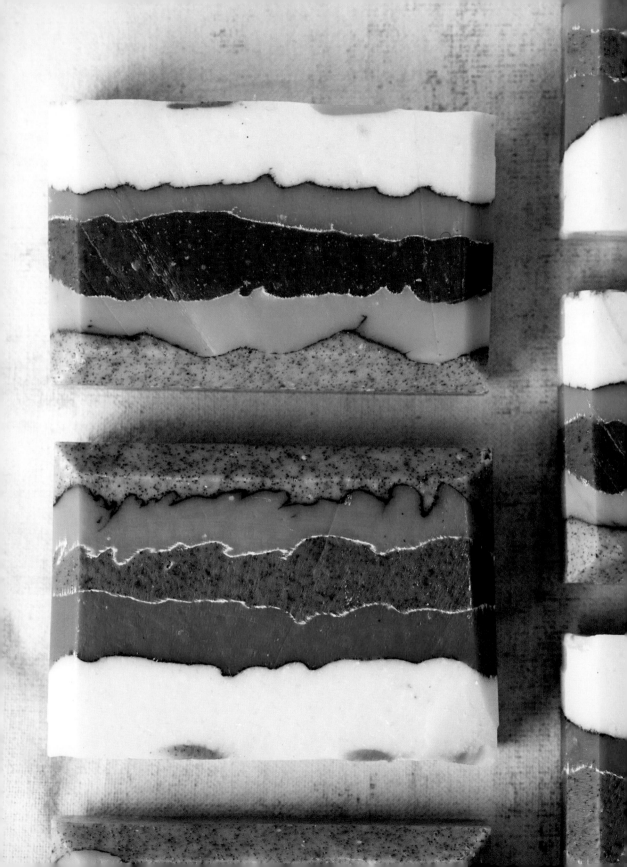

Layered Mica Lines
with Almond Milk

100% REPLACEMENT • MAKES 8 BARS

These bars have a lot going on, with a variety of textures in five different layers separated by mica lines. Almond flour and walnut shell powder provide gentle exfoliation. The addition of palm kernel flakes makes a hard bar and speeds up trace for pouring even layers.

Mold and Special Tools

10-inch (25 cm) silicone loaf mold
Fine-mesh strainer
5 easy-pour containers
2 powder dusters
Chopstick
Soap beveller (optional)

Oil Amounts

11.5 ounces/326 g coconut oil (35%)
9.9 ounces/281 g palm oil (30%)
3.3 ounces/94 g sweet almond oil (10%)
3.3 ounces/94 g shea butter (10%)
3.3 ounces/94 g palm kernel flakes (10%)
1.6 ounces/45 g castor oil (5%)

Lye Mixture

10.9 ounces/309 g almond milk, frozen (see page 8)
5.0 ounces/142 g lye (3% superfat)
3 teaspoons/15 mL sodium lactate

Fragrance Oil

2.4 ounces/68 g Neroli and Shea Blossom

Essential Oil Alternative

1.6 ounces/45 g lavender 40/42
0.8 ounce/23 g patchouli

Colorants

Disperse the first three into 1 tablespoon/15 mL sweet almond oil each.

1 teaspoon/5 mL brown oxide

1 teaspoon/5 mL titanium dioxide
¾ teaspoon/3.7 mL Neon Blue Raspberry pigment mixed with ¼ teaspoon/1.2 mL Zippy Blue pigment
2 teaspoons/10 mL Gold Sparkle mica
2 teaspoons/10 mL Cappuccino mica

Natural Colorant Alternative

Substitute the blue colorant with dispersed ultramarine blue at the same usage rates.

Additives

2 tablespoons/30 mL almond flour (see page 10)
2 tablespoons/30 mL walnut shell powder, divided

Safe Soaping!

Wear proper safety gear the whole time · Work in a well-ventilated space · No distractions

Use Any Milk

As with all these recipes, you can substitute any other kind of milk or dairy product, used in the same amount.

Make the Soap Batter

1 Melt the palm oil in its original container, mix it thoroughly, and measure it into a heatproof bowl large enough to hold the entire recipe. Melt and measure the coconut oil and add it to the bowl. Add the palm kernel flakes and shea butter to the hot oils and stir until melted. If needed, microwave the bowl in 10-second bursts to melt the butter completely. Add the sweet almond oil and castor oil and set the bowl aside.

2 Measure the frozen milk and the lye into separate heatproof containers. Slowly add the lye to the milk a tablespoon (15 mL) at a time, stirring continuously until all the lye has fully dissolved. This can take up to 30 minutes due to the cold temperature. Add the sodium lactate to the lye mixture and stir to combine.

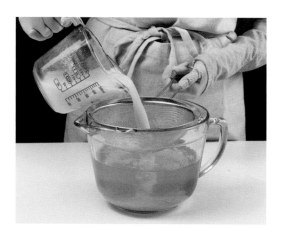

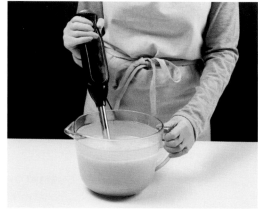

3 When the oils have cooled to between 100 and 105°F (38–40.5°C) and the lye mixture is between 75 and 85°F (24–29°C), gently pour the lye mixture through the strainer into the oils, stirring any residue gently with a spatula.

4 Insert the stick blender into the batter, tilting it so that any trapped air can escape. *Do not turn on the stick blender until the blades are fully immersed.* Alternate pulsing and stirring with the stick blender until a medium/thin trace is achieved. Add the fragrance oil to the batter and stir it in by hand.

Color the Soap

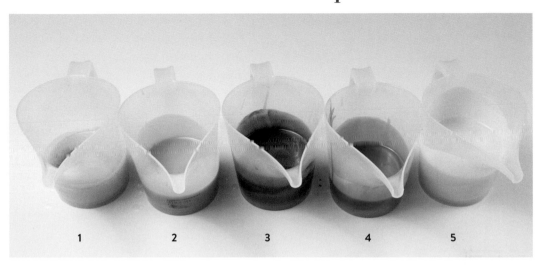

5 Add the following amounts of batter and colors to the containers, mixing them all in by hand:

- Container 1: A little more than 6.7 ounces (190 g) batter + 1 tablespoon (15 mL) walnut shell powder
- Container 2: A little more than 6.7 ounces (190 g) batter + ¼ teaspoon (1.2 mL) blue colorant
- Container 3: A little more than 10 ounces (283 g) batter + ¼ teaspoon (1.2 mL) brown colorant + 1 tablespoon (15 mL) walnut shell powder
- Container 4: A little more than 6.7 ounces (190 g) batter + ¾ teaspoon (3.7 mL) blue colorant
- Container 5: A little more than 13 ounces (369 g) batter + 1 teaspoon (5 mL) white colorant + 2 tablespoons (30 mL) almond flour

TECHNIQUE TIPS

- It can help to pour each layer slowly over the back of a spatula to keep the layers from breaking through.

- Between layers, give each container a quick stir to keep the batters from setting up too much.

- If the mica lines are too thick, the layers might separate once the loaf is cut; keep them thin and even.

Pour the Soap

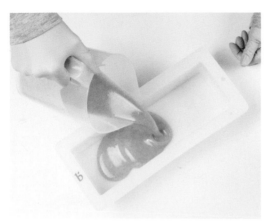

6 Pour the layers in the following order, each time tapping the mold against the counter to flatten the soap before sprinkling on the mica. Start with all of container 1 (plain batter with walnut shell powder).

- Plain
- Lighter blue
- Brown
- Darker blue
- White
- Reserved brown and blue

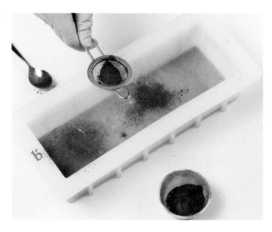

7 Gently tap 1 teaspoon (5 mL) of cappuccino mica across the surface.

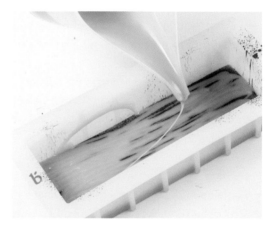

8 Next pour all of container 2 (lighter blue batter).

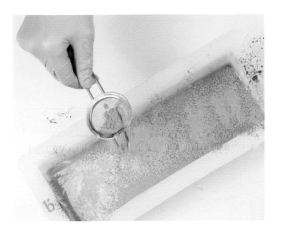

9 Dust with 1 teaspoon (5 mL) of Gold Sparkle mica.

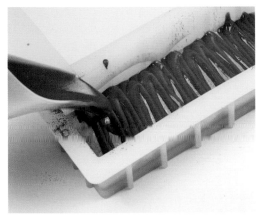

10 Pour most of container 3 (brown batter); reserve a couple spoonfuls for the top design.

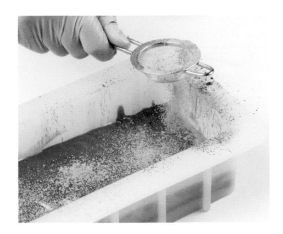

11 Dust with a thin layer of Gold Sparkle mica.

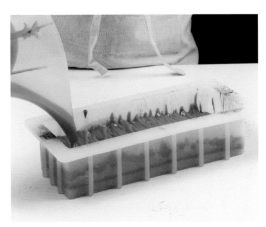

12 Pour most of container 4 (darker blue batter); reserve a couple spoonfuls for the top design.

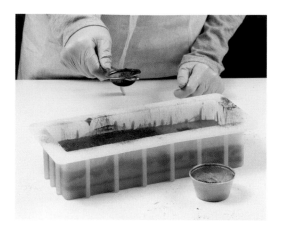

13 Dust evenly with a thin layer of Cappuccino mica.

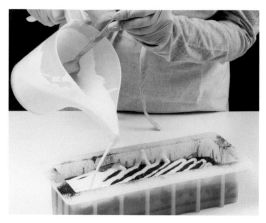

14 Pour all of container 5 (white batter).

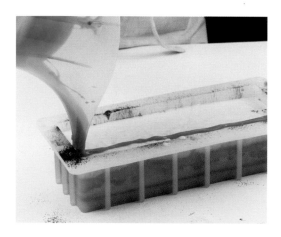

15 Use the reserved brown and blue batter to make two thin lines down the length of the mold, about a third of the way in from the sides.

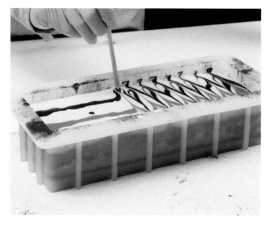

16 Insert a chopstick slightly into the top layer at one corner of the mold. Move the chopstick from side to side across the width of the mold to create the top design.

Final Steps

Spray thoroughly with 99% rubbing alcohol several times over 90 minutes to prevent soda ash. Let sit at room temperature for at least 48 hours before unmolding.

Cut the loaf on its side to avoid dragging the mica lines down the bars. Bevel the edges, if desired.

Let the bars cure in a well-ventilated area for 4 to 6 weeks before using, turning them every few days to ensure they cure evenly.

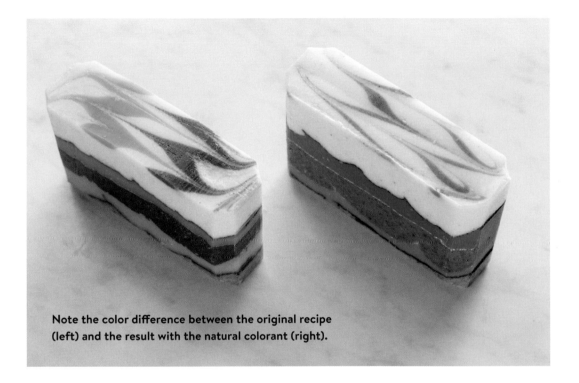

Note the color difference between the original recipe (left) and the result with the natural colorant (right).

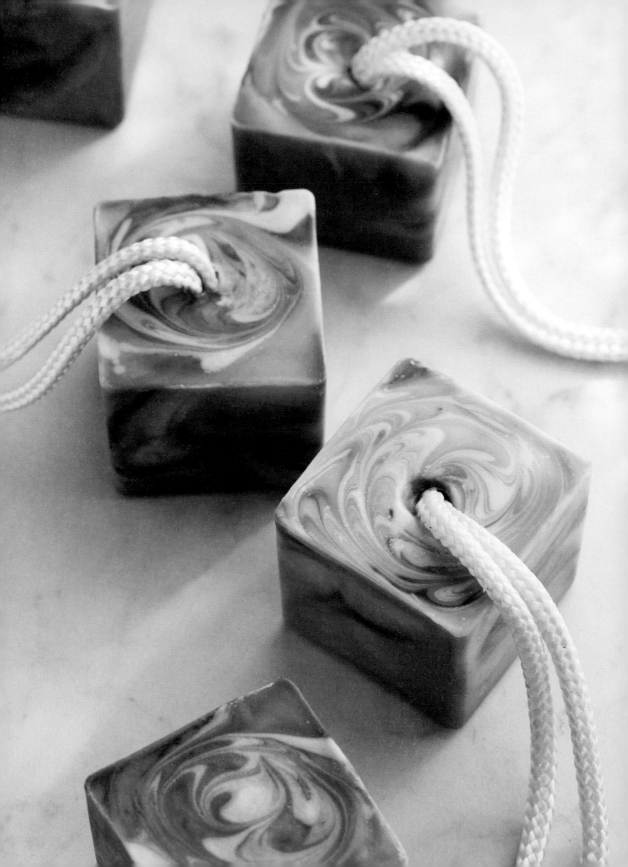

Cubed Swirls
with Almond Milk and Honey

100% REPLACEMENT • MAKES 9 BARS

Soap on a rope isn't just a throwback; it's useful! This recipe's almond milk creates an interesting base for the lovely almond and honey scent. The cube-shaped soaps also use honey to create a wonderful lather.

Mold and Special Tools

9-cube silicone mold
Fine-mesh strainer
3 easy-pour containers
9 white soap ropes (optional)
Several chopsticks

Oil Amounts

11.1 ounces/315 g
    coconut oil (30%)
11.1 ounces/315 g
    palm oil (30%)
9.2 ounces/261 g
    sweet almond oil (25%)
1.8 ounces/51 g
    shea butter (5%)
1.8 ounces/51 g
    kokum butter (5%)
1.8 ounces/51 g
    castor oil (5%)

Lye Mixture

12.2 ounces/346 g
    almond milk, frozen
5.4 ounces/153 g
    lye (3% superfat)
1 tablespoon/15 mL
    sodium lactate

Fragrance Oil Blend

0.7 ounce/20 g
    Almond Cybilla
2.0 ounces/57 g
    Pure Honey

Essential Oil Alternative

2.5 ounces/71 g
    patchouli

Colorants

Disperse each into 1 table-spoon/15 mL sweet almond oil.

1 teaspoon/5 mL
    yellow oxide
1 teaspoon/5 mL
    brown oxide
1 teaspoon/5 mL
    titanium dioxide

Additive

1 tablespoon/15 mL
    honey

Safe Soaping!

Wear proper safety gear the whole time · Work in a well-ventilated space · No distractions

Use Any Milk

As with all these recipes, you can substitute any other kind of milk or dairy product, used in the same amount.

Prepare Ahead

Make the almond milk according to the instructions on page 8; freeze. If you use commercial almond milk, choose an unflavored one with as few additives as possible.

Make the Soap Batter

1 Melt the palm oil in its original container, mix it thoroughly, and measure it into a heatproof bowl large enough to hold the entire recipe. Melt and measure the coconut oil and add it to the bowl. Add the shea butter and kokum butter to the hot oils and stir until melted. If needed, microwave the bowl in 10-second bursts to melt the butter completely. Add the sweet almond oil and castor oil and set the bowl aside.

2 Measure the frozen milk and the lye into separate heatproof containers. Slowly add the lye to the milk a tablespoon (15 mL) at a time, stirring continuously until all the lye has fully dissolved. This can take up to 30 minutes due to the cold temperature. Add the sodium lactate to the lye mixture and stir to combine.

3 When the oils have cooled to between 100 and 105°F (38–40.5°C) and the lye mixture is between 75 and 85°F (24–29°C), gently pour the lye mixture through the strainer into the oils, stirring any residue gently with a spatula.

4 Insert the stick blender into the batter, tilting it so that any trapped air can escape. *Do not turn on the stick blender until the blades are fully immersed.* Alternate pulsing and stirring with the stick blender until you reach emulsion.

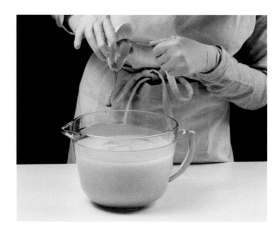

5 Add the honey and stick-blend until incorporated, keeping trace thin. Don't overblend.

Color the Soap

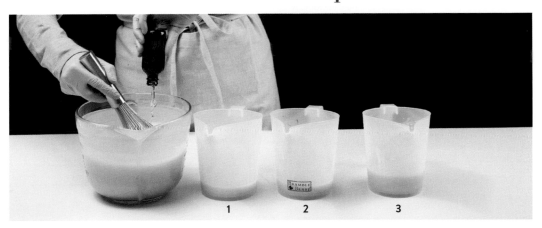

6 Pour the following amounts of batter into the easy-pour containers. Leave the remainder of the batter in the bowl and add a splash of the Pure Honey fragrance oil, whisking well.
- Container 1: 3.4 ounces (96 g) batter
- Container 2: 3.4 ounces (96 g) batter
- Container 3: 6.8 ounces (193 g) batter

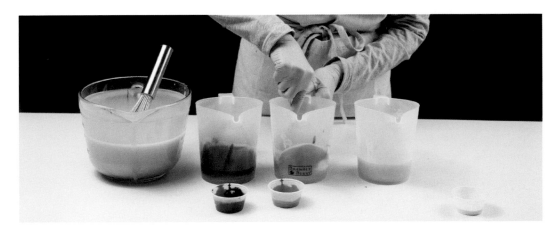

7 Add fragrance and colorants into the easy-pour containers as follows, whisking well to mix each color.
- Container 1: 1 teaspoon (5 mL) dispersed brown oxide + half the Almond Cybilla fragrance oil
- Container 2: 1 teaspoon (5 mL) dispersed yellow oxide + remaining Almond Cybilla fragrance oil
- Container 3: 2 teaspoons (10 mL) dispersed titanium dioxide + the rest of the Pure Honey fragrance oil

Swirl and Pour

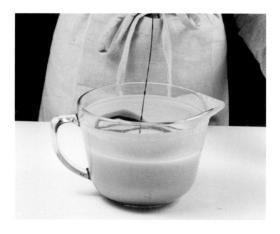

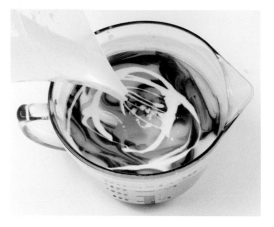

8 One at a time, pour the colored batters into the uncolored batter. Reserve a few spoonfuls of the white batter for the top swirl.

9 Pour from higher up and in a circular motion so that the colored batter breaks through and mixes into the uncolored batter.

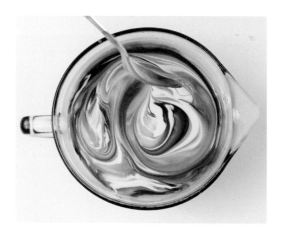

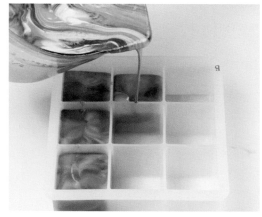

10 Stir the bowl just once with a spatula to swirl the three colors into the main batter. Do not overmix.

11 Pour the batter into the mold.

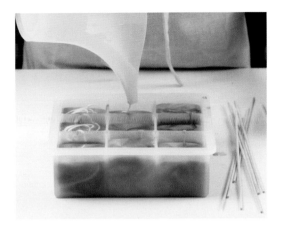

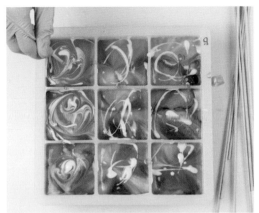

12 Top each cavity with a little of the reserved white batter and swirl it with a chopstick.

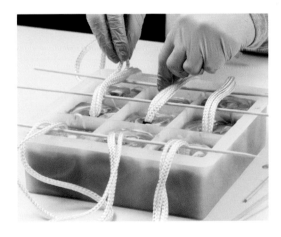

13 If using soap ropes, insert them into the center of each cavity until the black end cap just disappears into the soap batter. Use chopsticks to prop up the ropes.

Final Steps

Spray thoroughly with 99% rubbing alcohol several times over 90 minutes to prevent soda ash. Let sit at room temperature for at least 48 hours before unmolding. If the soaps are difficult to remove, wait another 24 hours. Do not try to remove the soaps by pulling on the ropes, as they will most likely come out of the fresh soap.

Let the bars cure in a well-ventilated area for 4 to 6 weeks before using, turning them every few days to ensure they cure evenly. **Note:** Swirls with the Almond Cybilla fragrance oil will darken as the soap cures.

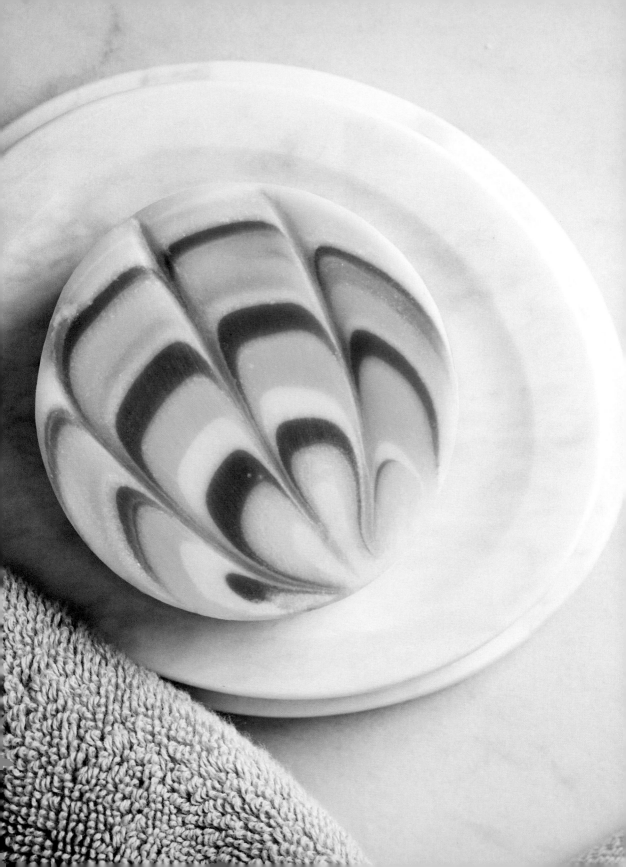

Round Peacock Swirl
with Goat's Milk

This recipe is a take on the elegant peacock swirl, which is usually done in a flat horizontal mold. Here we use a single-cavity silicone mold for a different shape, as well as squirt bottles and a chopstick to achieve the striking design. Because of the intricacy of the design, this recipe uses slow-moving oils. An extra boost of vitamin E helps slow trace and provides antioxidants.

Mold and Special Tools

12-bar round silicone mold
Fine-mesh strainer
4 easy-pour containers
4 squirt bottles
Cutting board for moving
    mold to freezer
Chopstick

Oil Amounts

9.9 ounces/281 g
    pure olive oil (30%)
6.6 ounces/187 g
    avocado oil (20%)
3.3 ounces/94 g
    coconut oil (10%)
3.3 ounces/94 g
    palm oil (10%)
3.3 ounces/94 g
    apricot kernel oil (10%)

3.3 ounces/94 g
    avocado butter (10%)
1.6 ounces/45 g
    shea butter (5%)
1.6 ounces/45 g
    castor oil (5%)

Lye Mixture

10.8 ounces/306 g
    goat's milk, frozen
4.4 ounces/125 g
    lye (3% superfat)
3 teaspoons/15 mL
    sodium lactate

Fragrance Oil

2.4 ounces/68 g
    Cactus Flower

Essential Oil Alternative

1.8 ounces/51 g
    tangerine
0.6 ounce/17 g
    elemi

Colorants

Disperse each into 1 table-spoon/15 mL apricot kernel oil.

1 teaspoon/5 mL
    Yellow mica
1 teaspoon/5 mL
    Raspberry mica
1 teaspoon/5 mL
    Kermit Green mica

Natural Colorant Alternative

Replace the micas with dispersed ultramarine pink oxide, yellow oxide, and green oxide at the same usage rates.

Additive

0.5 ounce/14 g vitamin E oil

Safe Soaping!

Wear proper safety gear the whole time · Work in a well-ventilated space · No distractions

Use Any Milk

As with all these recipes, you can substitute any other kind of milk or dairy product, used in the same amount.

Make the Soap Batter

1 Melt the palm oil in its original container, mix it thoroughly, and measure it into a heatproof bowl large enough to hold the entire recipe. Melt and measure the coconut oil and add it to the bowl. Add the avocado butter and shea butter to the hot oils and stir until melted. If needed, microwave the bowl in 10-second bursts to melt the butter completely. Add the apricot kernel oil, avocado oil, olive oil, and castor oil and set the bowl aside.

2 Measure the frozen milk and the lye into separate heatproof containers. Slowly add the lye to the milk a tablespoon (15 mL) at a time, stirring continuously until all the lye has fully dissolved. This can take up to 30 minutes due to the cold temperature. Add the sodium lactate to the lye mixture and stir to combine.

3 When the oils have cooled to between 100 and 105°F (38–40.5°C) and the lye mixture is between 75 and 85°F (24–29°C), gently pour the lye mixture through the strainer into the oils, stirring any residue gently with a spatula.

4 Insert the stick blender into the batter, tilting it so that any trapped air can escape. *Do not turn on the stick blender until the blades are fully immersed.* Alternate pulsing and stirring with the stick blender until a very thin trace is achieved.

5 Whisk in the vitamin E and fragrance oils.

Color and Pour

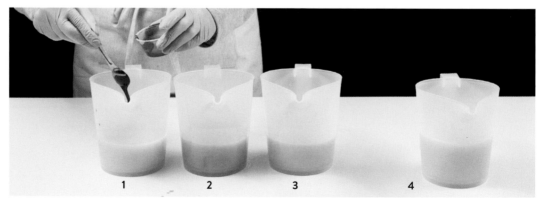

6 Pour the batter into the easy-pour containers in the following amounts, stirring in the colorants by hand.

- Container 1: 10 ounces (283 g) batter + 1 teaspoon (5 mL) dispersed Raspberry mica
- Container 2: 10 ounces (283 g) batter + 1 teaspoon (5 mL) dispersed Kermit Green mica
- Container 3: 10 ounces (283 g) batter + 1 teaspoon (5 mL) dispersed Yellow mica
- Container 4: 17 ounces (482 g) batter, uncolored

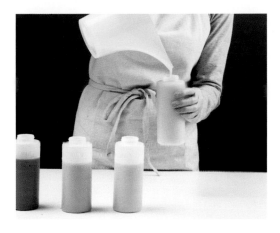

7 Pour each color into its own squirt bottle.

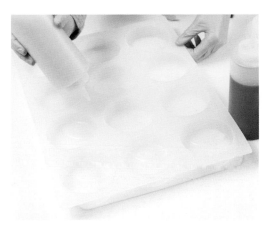

8 Place the mold on top of the cutting board for support and squirt a dot of white soap batter along one side of each cavity. You don't want to cover the entire bottom; the batter will spread on its own as you add more layers.

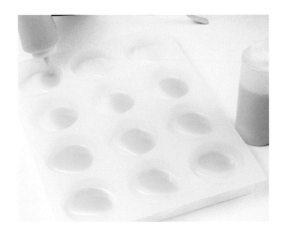

9 Squirt a dot of another color batter in the same spot, on top of the first.

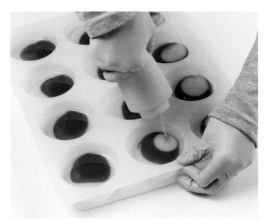

10 Alternate colors, always squirting into the same spot in each cavity. There is more plain batter than colored, so use it more often. Tap the mold and cutting board on the counter when needed to even out the batter, as it will start to pool up wherever you squirt batter in.

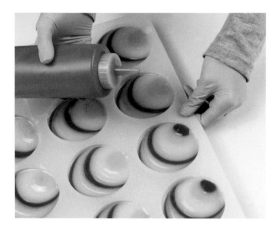

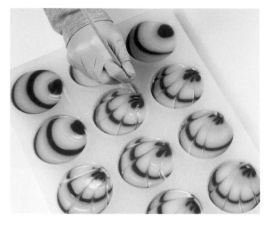

11 Repeat until you are out of batter, making smaller dots as you near the bottom of the cavities.

12 Insert the chopstick to the bottom of the cavity and draw lines from the outer edges of the cavities toward the bottom dot (see diagram). Make four or five lines per circle. Wipe the chopstick clean after every pass for smooth lines.

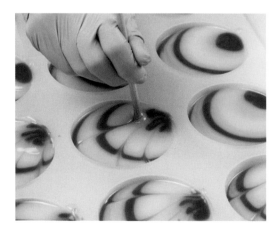

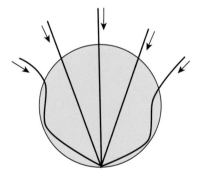

Final Steps

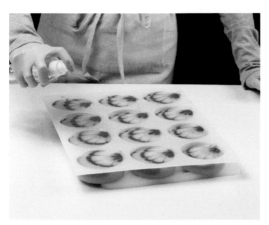

13 Spray thoroughly with 99% rubbing alcohol several times over 90 minutes to prevent soda ash. Let sit for at least 48 hours at room temperature before unmolding.

14 Let the bars cure in a well-ventilated area for 4 to 6 weeks before using, turning them every few days to ensure they cure evenly.

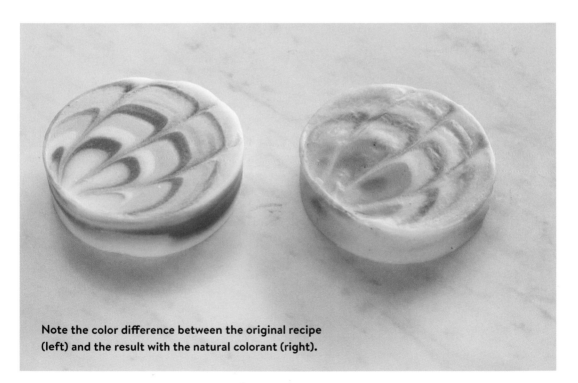

Note the color difference between the original recipe (left) and the result with the natural colorant (right).

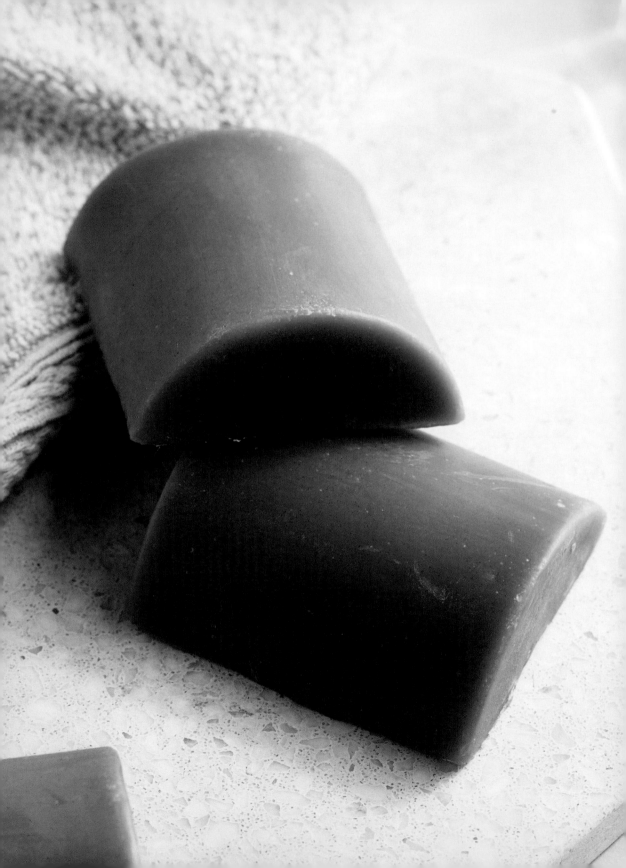

Shampoo Bars *with Hemp*
Milk and Apple Cider Vinegar

25% ADDED AT TRACE • MAKES 6 BARS

Homemade shampoo bars are not for everyone; it may take a few washes to get used to the decreased lather. This luxurious bar is loaded with skin- and hair-loving oils like hempseed, wheat germ, argan, chia, neem, and jojoba. To make it a shampoo bar, it also contains apple cider vinegar to help prevent buildup of oil and skin cells on the scalp and bring down the pH, making it gentle on the scalp. The essential oils impart a wonderful citrusy-minty aroma. The color of the bars comes from the natural colors of the different oils. These bars go in the freezer overnight to prevent overheating.

Mold and Special Tools
Half-round silicone mold
Cutting board for moving
  mold to freezer

Oil Amounts
2.4 ounces/68 g
  coconut oil (15%)
1.9 ounces/54 g
  babassu oil (12%)
1.6 ounces/45 g
  sweet almond oil (10%)
1.6 ounces/45 g
  avocado oil (10%)
1.6 ounces/45 g
  hempseed oil (10%)
1.6 ounces/45 g
  pure olive oil (10%)
1.3 ounces/37 g
  castor oil (8%)

0.8 ounce/23 g
  wheat germ oil (5%)
0.8 ounce/23 g
  argan oil (5%)
0.8 ounce/23 g
  chia seed oil (5%)
0.8 ounce/23 g
  jojoba oil (5%)
0.8 ounce/23 g
  neem oil (5%)

Lye-Water
2.6 ounces/74 g
  distilled water
2.2 ounces/62 g
  lye (3% superfat)
1 teaspoon/5 mL
  sodium lactate

Essential Oil Blend
0.4 ounce/11 g
  blue chamomile
0.3 ounce/8.5 g
  lemongrass
0.2 ounce/6 g
  peppermint 1st distilled
0.1 ounce/2.8 g
  Atlas cedarwood

Additives
1.3 ounces/37 g
  hemp milk
0.8 ounce/23 g
  nettle extract
1.3 ounces/37 g
  apple cider vinegar
0.8 ounce/23 g
  DL panthenol*

*Vitamin B_5; added for hair softening and conditioning

Safe Soaping!
Wear proper safety gear the whole time · Work in a well-ventilated space · No distractions

Use Any Milk
As with all these recipes, you can substitute any other kind of milk or dairy product, used in the same amount.

Prepare Ahead

Make the hemp milk according to the instructions on page 8.

Measure out and dissolve the panthenol into the apple cider vinegar.

Place the mold on the cutting board.

Make the Soap Batter

1 Melt the babassu oil in its original container and measure it into a heatproof
bowl large enough to hold the entire recipe.
Melt and measure the coconut oil and add it
to the bowl. Add the argan oil, avocado oil,
castor oil, chia seed oil, hempseed oil, jojoba
oil, neem oil, olive oil, sweet almond oil, and
wheat germ oil and set the bowl aside.

2 Measure the distilled water and the lye
into separate heatproof containers. Add
the lye to the water a tablespoon (15 mL) at
a time (never add the liquid to the lye). Stir
continuously until the lye fully dissolves and
the water becomes clear. Stir the sodium
lactate into the lye-water.

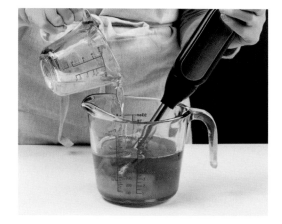

3 When the oils and the lye-water have
cooled to about 105°F (40.5°C), add the
lye-water to the oils, pouring it over the shaft
of the stick blender to minimize air bubbles.

4 Insert the stick blender into the batter, tilting it so that any trapped air can
escape. *Do not turn on the stick blender until the
blades are fully immersed.* Alternate pulsing and
stirring with the stick blender until emulsified.

Mix and Pour

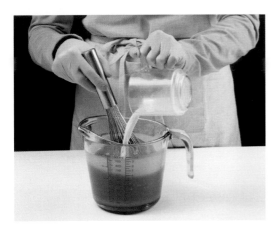

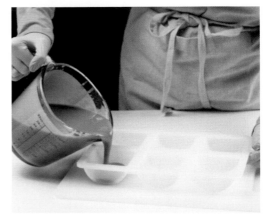

5 Add the nettle extract, hemp milk, and essential oils and whisk briefly to combine. Stay at a thin trace.

6 Add the apple cider vinegar (this will quickly start to thicken the batter). Blend just until well mixed, then pour the batter into the mold. Smooth and flatten the batter with a spatula.

Final Steps

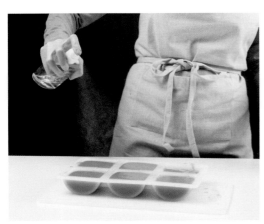

7 Spray thoroughly with 99% rubbing alcohol several times over 90 minutes to prevent soda ash. Place the mold in the freezer overnight.

8 Remove the mold from the freezer and let sit for 48 hours before unmolding. Frozen soaps tend to soften quite a bit as they thaw and need time to harden again.

9 Let the bars cure in a well-ventilated area for 4 to 6 weeks before using, turning them every few days to ensure they cure evenly.

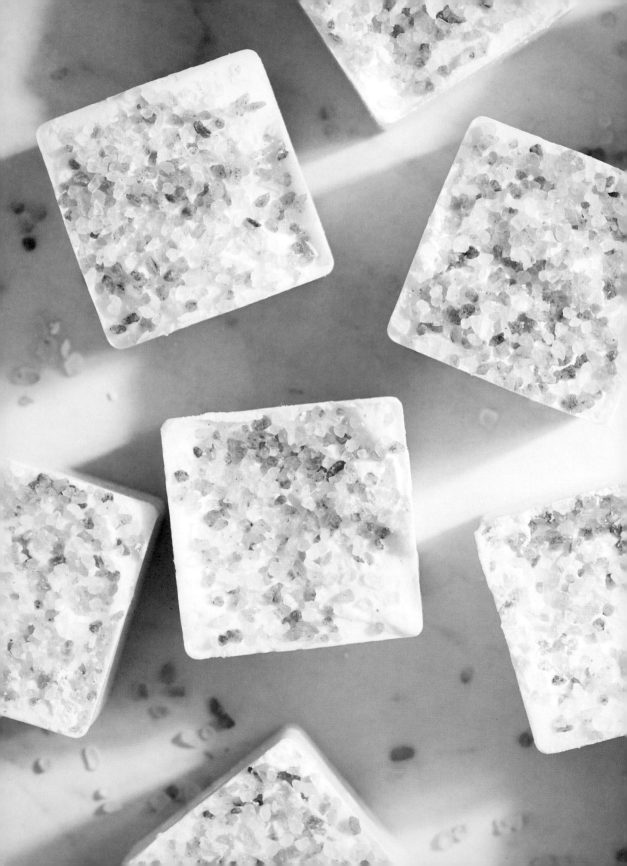

Pink Himalayan *and* Dendritic Salt Bars
with Flax Milk

30% ADDED AT TRACE • MAKES 9 BARS

This is a classic salt bar with the unusual addition of flax milk. Salt is an incredible hardening agent and creates a mineral-rich bar of soap. Dendritic salt is nonclumping, making it easier to mix into the soap batter. Because salt inhibits lather, this recipe compensates by using extra coconut oil. The pink Himalayan sea salt accent contrasts beautifully with the crisp white color of the bars.

Mold and Special Tools
9-cube silicone mold

Oil Amounts
21.6 ounces/612 g
  coconut oil (80%)
2.7 ounces/76 g
  sweet almond oil (10%)
1.3 ounces/37 g
  kokum butter (5%)
1.3 ounces/37 g
  castor oil (5%)

Lye-Water
6.3 ounces/179 g
  distilled water
3.8 ounces/108 g
  lye (15% superfat)

Essential Oil
1.0 ounce/28 g
  Egyptian geranium

Colorant
2 teaspoons/10 mL
  titanium dioxide
  dispersed into
  2 tablespoons/30 mL
  sweet almond oil

Additives
2.6 ounces/74 g
  flax milk
24 ounces/680 g
  dendritic salt
¼ cup/59 mL
  pink Himalayan sea salt,
  medium grind

Safe Soaping!
Wear proper safety gear the whole time · Work in a well-ventilated space · No distractions

Use Any Milk
As with all these recipes, you can substitute any other kind of milk or dairy product, used in the same amount.

Prepare Ahead

Make the flax milk according to the instructions on page 10.

Make the Soap Batter

1 Melt and measure the coconut oil into a heatproof bowl large enough to hold the entire recipe. Add the kokum butter to the hot coconut oil and stir until melted. If needed, microwave the bowl in 10-second bursts to melt the butter completely. Add the sweet almond oil and castor oil and set the bowl aside.

2 Measure the distilled water and the lye into separate heatproof containers. Add the lye to the water a tablespoon (15 mL) at a time (never add the liquid to the lye). Stir continuously until the lye fully dissolves and the water becomes clear. Stir the sodium lactate into the lye-water.

3 When the oils and the lye-water have cooled to about 105°F (40.5°C), add the lye-water to the oils, pouring it over the shaft of the stick blender to minimize air bubbles.

4 Insert the stick blender into the batter, tilting it so that any trapped air can escape. *Do not turn on the stick blender until the blades are fully immersed.* Alternate pulsing and stirring with the stick blender until a very thin trace is achieved.

Mix and Pour

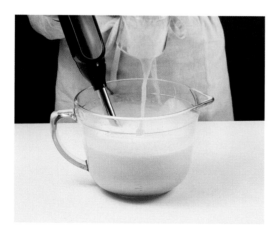

5 Add the flax milk, dispersed titanium dioxide, and essential oil and pulse the stick blender until incorporated, keeping trace light.

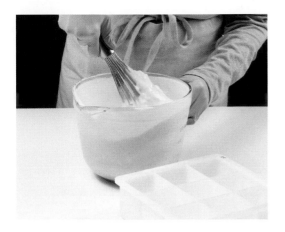

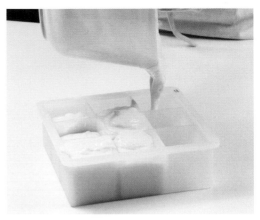

6 Add the dendritic salt and mix with a whisk to break up any clumps. This will quickly thicken up the batter, so be prepared to mix and pour once it has been added.

7 Pour or spoon the batter into the mold cavities, leaving a little room at the top of each for the pink sea salt.

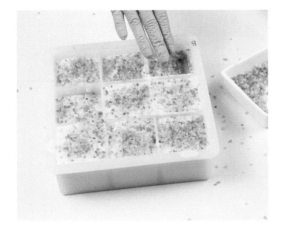

Final Steps

9 Set aside at room temperature to harden. Salt bars harden quickly and should be unmolded the same day. Check the bars after 3 or 4 hours, waiting another 1 or 2 hours, if needed. Leaving the bars in the mold too long will make them brittle and difficult to remove, resulting in crumbly soaps.

10 Let the bars cure in a well-ventilated area for 4 to 6 weeks before using, turning them every few days to ensure they cure evenly.

8 Sprinkle sea salt on top of each cavity until completely covered. Gently push the salt in with your gloved finger so that it sticks in the batter and won't fall out when unmolded.

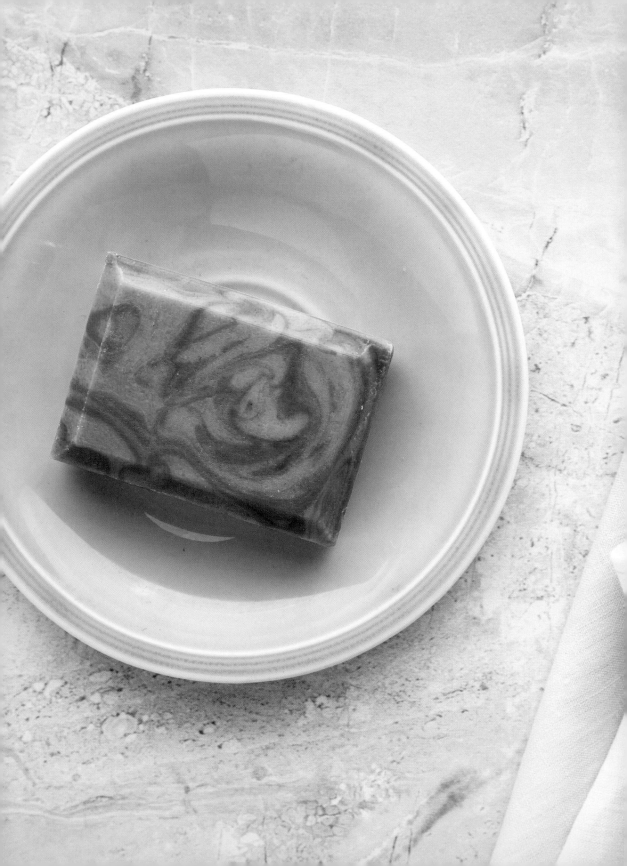

Super Rainbow Swirl

100% Replacement • Makes 16 Bars

This palm-free recipe uses vibrant colors and six in-the-pot swirls to make a rainbow swirl design. It is an advanced recipe that contains lots of slow-moving liquid oils to give time to achieve good results. This recipe is designed for use with an undivided horizontal mold; a special cutting technique reveals the inside of the bars.

Mold and Special Tools

9-bar birchwood mold
    with silicone liner
Fine-mesh strainer
6 easy-pour containers
Chopstick for swirling tops
    (optional)
Wire soap slicer
Soap beveller (optional)

Oil Amounts

16.5 ounces/468 g
    coconut oil (25%)
13.2 ounces/374 g
    sweet almond oil (20%)
13.2 ounces/374 g
    pure olive oil (20%)
13.2 ounces/374 g
    canola oil (20%)
6.6 ounces/187 g
    sunflower seed oil (10%)
3.3 ounces/94 g
    castor oil (5%)

Lye Mixture

21.7 ounces/615 g
    2% milk, frozen
9.0 ounces/255 g lye
    (6% superfat)
2 tablespoons/30 mL
    sodium lactate

Fragrance Oil

4.8 ounces/136 g
    Electric Lemonade
    Cocktail

Essential Oil Alternative

3.2 ounces/91 g
    grapefruit
1.6 ounces/45 g
    lavender 40/42

Colorants

Disperse each in 1 tablespoon/ 15 mL of sweet almond oil.

1 teaspoon/5 mL
    Electric Bubblegum
    pigment

1 teaspoon/5 mL
    Nuclear Orange pigment
1 teaspoon/5 mL
    Fizzy Lemonade pigment
1 teaspoon/5 mL
    Zippy Blue pigment
1 teaspoon/5 mL
    Radiant Plum pigment
¼ teaspoon/1.2 mL
    Zippy Blue + ¾ teaspoon/
    3.7 mL Fizzy Lemonade

Natural Colorant Alternative

Replace the colorants with dispersed ultramarine pink pigment, yellow oxide, green oxide, ultramarine blue oxide, and ultramarine violet pigment at the same usage rates.

Safe Soaping!

Wear proper safety gear the whole time · Work in a well-ventilated space · No distractions

Use Any Milk

As with all these recipes, you can substitute any other kind of milk or dairy product, used in the same amount.

Make the Soap Batter

1 Melt and measure the coconut oil into a heatproof bowl large enough to hold the entire recipe. Add the olive oil, sweet almond oil, canola oil, sunflower seed oil, and castor oil and set the bowl aside.

2 Measure the frozen milk and the lye into separate heatproof containers. Slowly add the lye to the milk a tablespoon (15 mL) at a time, stirring continuously until all the lye has fully dissolved. This can take up to 30 minutes due to the cold temperature. Add the sodium lactate to the lye mixture and stir to combine.

3 When the oils have cooled to between 100 and 105°F (38–40.5°C) and the lye mixture is between 75 and 85°F (24–29°C), gently pour the lye mixture through the strainer into the oils, stirring any residue gently with a spatula.

4 Insert the stick blender into the batter, tilting it so that any trapped air can escape. *Do not turn on the stick blender until the blades are fully immersed.* Alternate pulsing and stirring with the stick blender until a thin trace is achieved.

5 Add the fragrance oil and mix in by hand.

Color and Swirl

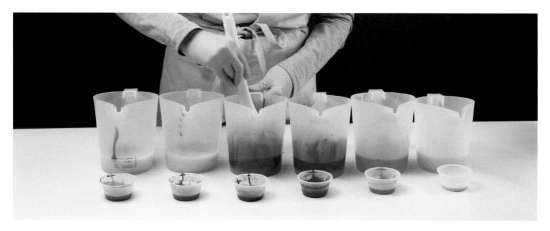

6 Pour 6 ounces (170 g) of soap batter into each easy-pour container (this will leave you with more than half the batter). Add one teaspoon of dispersed colorant to each container and mix well by hand.

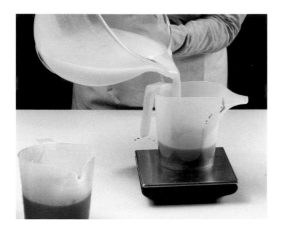

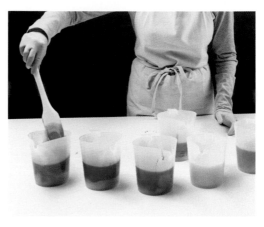

7 Divide the remaining batter equally among the six containers (about 10 ounces/283 g each) by pouring it from different heights and in a circular motion so that it swirls into the colored batters.

8 Give each container a single stir to slightly combine the colors. Do not overmix.

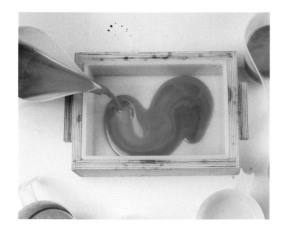

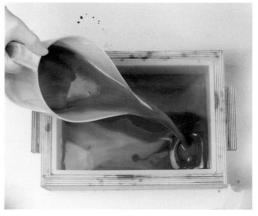

9 Pour the colors into the mold, adding a little of each color at a time in different areas, from different heights, using different patterns. This is the fun and creative part; there are no exact measurements or particular order.

Tap the mold on the table after every few passes to release any air bubbles. Keep pouring until the mold is as full as possible.

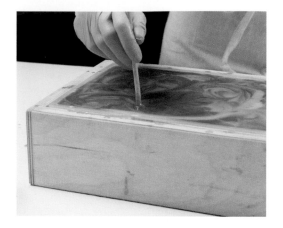

10 Leave the top as is or slightly insert a chopstick into the topmost layer and lightly swirl to add more of a design.

Final Steps

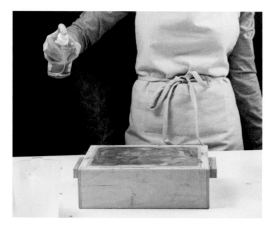

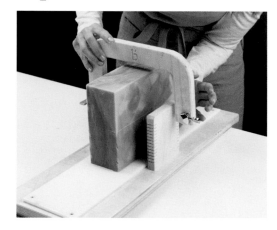

11 Tap the mold on the table one more time. Spray thoroughly with 99% rubbing alcohol several times over 90 minutes to prevent soda ash. Let the mold sit at room temperature for 48 hours before unmolding.

12 When the soap has hardened, remove it from the liner. Cut it in half lengthwise to make two rectangular loaves.

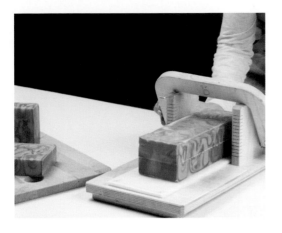

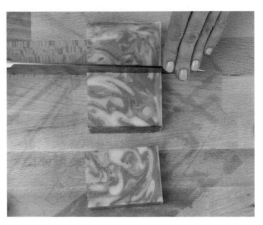

13 Slice each loaf lengthwise through the center to reveal the swirl inside.

14 Cut each loaf into four individual bars. Optional: bevel the edges of each bar (8 sides per bar) to reveal more of the design.

15 Let the bars cure in a well-ventilated area for 4 to 6 weeks before using, turning them every few days so that they cure evenly.

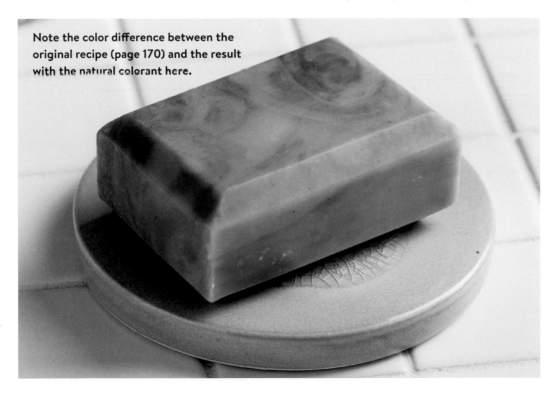

Note the color difference between the original recipe (page 170) and the result with the natural colorant here.

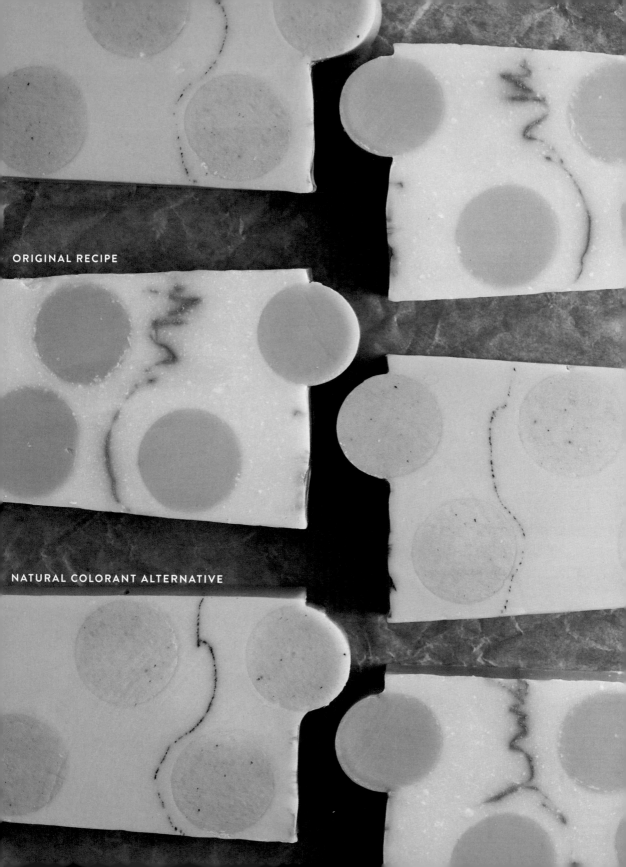

ORIGINAL RECIPE

NATURAL COLORANT ALTERNATIVE

Embedded Pencil Wave
with Donkey's Milk

100% REPLACEMENT • MAKES 10 BARS

Because it uses premade soap embeds in the design, this is a two-part recipe that takes at least two days to complete. The wave is achieved by incorporating a mica line at a thinner-than-usual trace. Bramble Berry's liquid silk (silk amino acids dissolved in water) added at 5% gives the bars a silky, smooth feel. A swirl of mica painted on top adds a final artistic touch. (Donkey's milk is fun to experiment with, but you can substitute any other kind of milk.)

STAGE 1: MAKE THE EMBEDS

Molds and Special Tools
4 mini round silicone
    column molds
Fine-mesh strainer
2 easy-pour containers
4 rubber bands to hold molds

Oil Amounts
4.5 ounces/128 g
    coconut oil (30%)
4.5 ounces/128 g
    palm oil (30%)
4.5 ounces/128 g
    apricot kernel oil (30%)
0.7 ounce/20 g
    shea butter (5%)
0.7 ounce/20 g
    castor oil (5%)

Lye Mixture
4.9 ounces/139 g
    donkey's milk, frozen
2.1 ounces/60 g
    lye (7% superfat)
1 teaspoon/5 mL
    sodium lactate

Fragrance Oil
1.1 ounces/31 g
    Energy

Essential Oil Alternative
0.5 ounce/14 g
    lemon
0.5 ounce/14 g
    Valencia orange

Colorant
1 teaspoon/5 mL
    Sunset Orange mica
    dispersed into 1 table-
    spoon/15 mL apricot
    kernel oil

Natural Colorant Alternative
3 teaspoons/15 mL
    ultramarine pink pigment

Additive
1.1 ounces/31 g
    Liquid Silk

Safe Soaping!
Wear proper safety gear the whole time · Work in a well-ventilated space · No distractions

Use Any Milk
As with all these recipes, you can substitute any other kind of milk or dairy product, used in the same amount.

Prepare Ahead

Assemble the four column molds, pressing along the edges to ensure the seals are closed tightly and there are no gaps. Bunch them together and secure with the rubber bands. Stand them upright in one of the easy-pour containers.

Make and Pour the Embed Batter

1 Melt the palm oil in its original container, mix it thoroughly, and measure it into a heatproof bowl large enough to hold the entire recipe. Melt and measure the coconut oil and add it to the bowl. Add the shea butter to the hot oils and stir until melted. If needed, microwave the bowl in 10-second bursts to melt the shea butter completely. Measure and add the apricot kernel oil and castor oil and set the bowl aside.

2 Measure the frozen milk and the lye into separate heatproof containers. Slowly add the lye to the milk a tablespoon (15 mL) at a time, stirring continuously until all the lye has fully dissolved. This can take up to 30 minutes due to the cold temperature. Add the sodium lactate to the lye mixture and stir to combine.

3 When the oils have cooled to between 100 and 105°F (38–40.5°C) and the lye mixture is between 75 and 85°F (24–29°C), gently pour the lye mixture through the strainer into the oils, stirring any residue gently with a spatula.

4 Insert the stick blender into the batter, tilting it so that any trapped air can escape. *Do not turn on the stick blender until the blades are fully immersed.* Alternate pulsing and stirring with the stick blender until a thin trace is achieved.

5 Add the fragrance oil, Liquid Silk, and 1 teaspoon (5 mL) of dispersed orange colorant to the batter and stick-blend to achieve light trace. (Save the rest of the colorant for stage 2.)

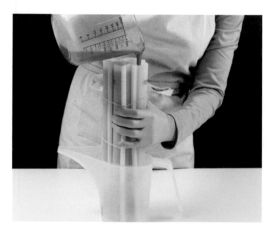

6 Pour the batter into the column molds and let sit at room temperature for 24 to 48 hours to harden before unmolding.

Mold and Special Tools

Tall 12-inch (30.5 cm)
silicone loaf mold
Fine-mesh strainer
Easy-pour container
Powder duster
3 chopsticks

Oil Amounts

6.6 ounces/187 g
coconut oil (30%)
6.6 ounces/187 g
palm oil (30%)
6.6 ounces/187 g
apricot kernel oil (30%)
1.1 ounces/31 g
shea butter (5%)
1.1 ounces/31 g
castor oil (5%)

Lye Mixture

7.2 ounces/204 g
donkey's milk, frozen
3.0 ounces/85 g lye
(7% superfat)
2 teaspoons/10 mL
sodium lactate

Fragrance Oil

1.6 ounces/45 g
Energy

Essential Oil Alternative

0.8 ounce/23 g
lemon
0.8 ounce/23 g
Valencia orange

Colorants

1 teaspoon/5 mL
Yellow mica dispersed
into 1 tablespoon/15 mL
apricot kernel oil
Remaining dispersed Sunset
Orange mica from Stage 1
Approximately 2 teaspoons/
10 mL Sunset Orange mica,
not dispersed, for pencil line

Natural Colorant Alternative

Replace the Yellow mica with
dispersed yellow oxide at the
same usage rate. Use ultramarine
pink pigment for the pencil line.

Additive

1.6 ounces/45 g
Liquid Silk

Make the Base Batter

1 Melt the palm oil in its original container, mix it thoroughly, and measure it into a heatproof bowl large enough to hold the entire recipe. Melt and measure the coconut oil and add it to the bowl. Add the shea butter to the hot oils and stir until melted. If needed, microwave the bowl in 10-second bursts to melt the shea butter completely. Add the apricot kernel oil and castor oil and set the bowl aside.

2 Measure the frozen milk and the lye into separate heatproof containers. Slowly add the lye to the milk a tablespoon (15 mL) at a time, stirring continuously until all the lye has fully dissolved. This can take up to 30 minutes due to the cold temperature. Add the sodium lactate to the lye mixture and stir to combine.

3 When the oils have cooled to between 100 and 105°F (38–40.5°C) and the lye mixture is between 75 and 85°F (24–29°C), gently pour the lye mixture through the strainer into the oils, stirring any residue gently with a spatula.

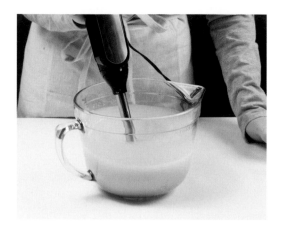

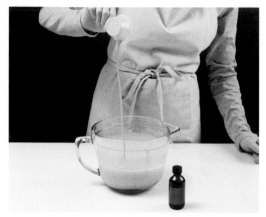

4 Insert the stick blender into the batter, tilting it so that any trapped air can escape. *Do not turn on the stick blender until the blades are fully immersed.* Alternate pulsing and stirring with the stick blender until a thin trace is achieved.

5 Add the fragrance oil, Liquid Silk, and the Yellow mica to the batter and stick-blend to combine. Keep trace light.

Pour and Embed

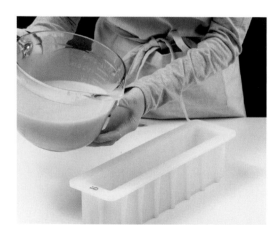

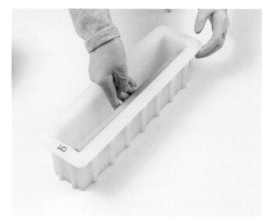

6 Pour just enough batter into the mold to fully cover the bottom of the mold.

7 Place an embed into the batter along one side of the mold.

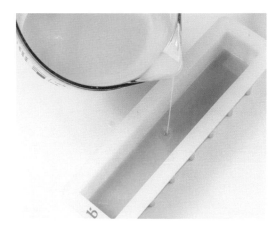

8 Pour just enough batter to fully cover the embed.

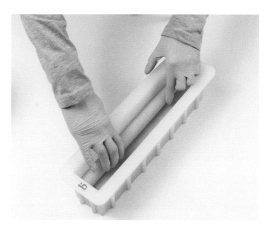

9 Place another embed into the mold on the opposite side of the first embed. Lay it down gently so that it doesn't sink down too far.

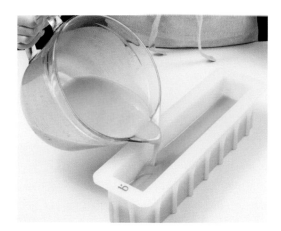

10 Again pour just enough batter to fully cover the embed. Pour the rest of the batter into an easy-pour container for easier pouring and layering.

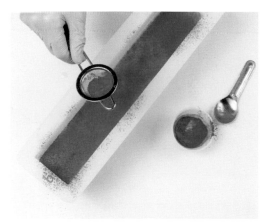

11 Place the Sunset Orange mica into the powder duster and gently tap it over the soap to create a light dusting of mica across the surface. Keep this layer thin or the soap may separate once sliced.

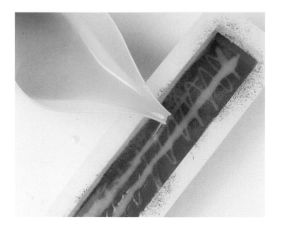 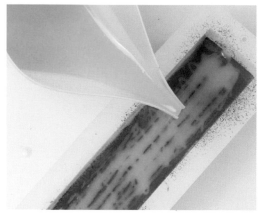

12 Carefully pour a layer of batter over the mica layer. Pour close to the surface, making very thin, long lines back and forth across the length and width of the mold. The thin trace will slightly disrupt the line. Keep pouring low and slow until the entire mica layer is covered.

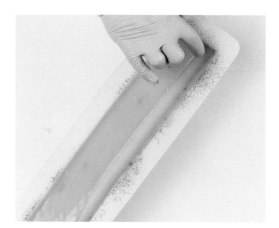 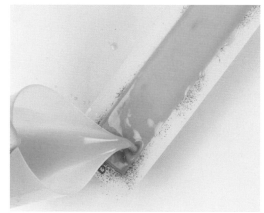

13 Place another embed into the mold on the same side as the first one. Let the embed sink down slightly into the batter, giving it a slight push if needed, to smooth and curve the mica line around the embed.

14 Pour the remaining yellow batter into the mold.

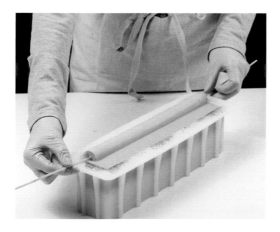

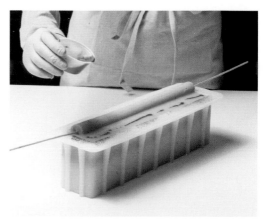

15 Poke a chopstick slightly into each end of the remaining embed and lay the embed halfway into the soap on the opposite side from the previous embed. The chopsticks will rest on the mold and hold the embed in place as the batter sets.

16 Drip the dispersed Sunset Orange mica along the yellow batter in an uneven pattern.

Final Steps

Lightly spray the tops with 99% rubbing alcohol to prevent soda ash. Spraying too much or too closely will cause the mica painting to bleed.

Let sit for 48 hours at room temperature before unmolding and cutting. Slice these bars on their sides to prevent the knife from making drag lines.

Let the bars cure in a well-ventilated area for 4 to 6 weeks before using, turning them every few days so that they cure evenly.

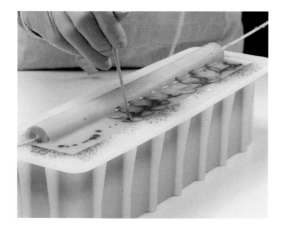

17 Use a chopstick to swirl the drops into a figure-eight pattern down the length of the mold.

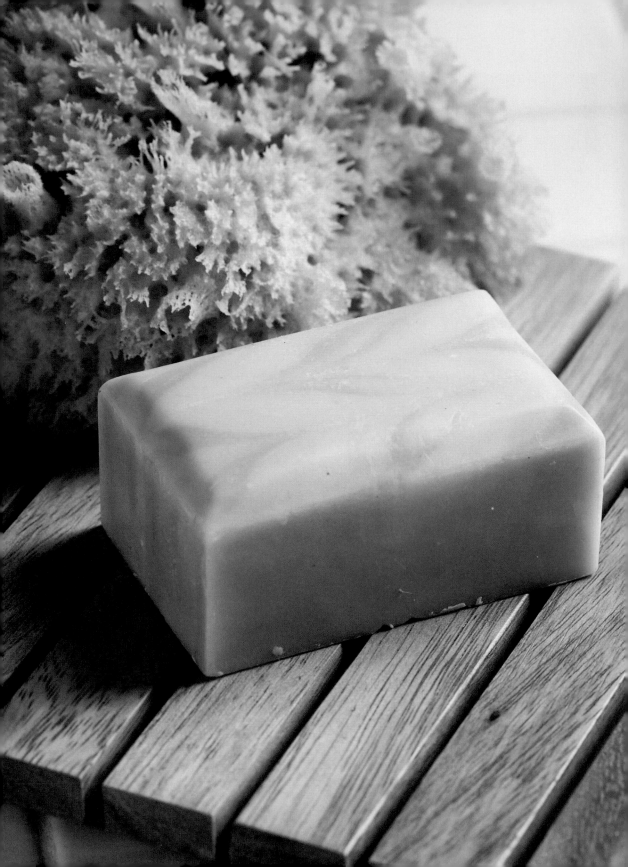

Linear Swirl
with Sour Cream

This gorgeous linear swirl is achieved in a flat mold using squirt bottles to make the lines and a chopstick for the final delicate touch. Dividers pull the design down the sides, adding interest to the entire bar. This recipe uses freshly made sour cream and vitamin E for extra pampering and skin resilience.

Mold and Special Tools

18-bar birchwood mold with silicone liner and dividers
2 extra bowls with spouts for mixing colors
3 squirt bottles
Chopstick for swirling
Soap beveller (optional)

Oil Amounts

27.7 ounces/785 g
pure olive oil (42%)
6.6 ounces/187 g
coconut oil (10%)
6.6 ounces/187 g
palm oil (10%)
6.6 ounces/187 g
avocado oil (10%)
6.6 ounces/187 g
hempseed oil (10%)
6.6 ounces/187 g
shea butter (10%)

3.3 ounces/94 g
sweet almond oil (5%)
2.0 ounces/57 g
castor oil (3%)

Lye-Water

15.2 ounces/431 g
distilled water
8.5 ounces/241 g
lye (7% superfat)
2 tablespoons/30 mL
sodium lactate

Fragrance Oil

4.8 ounces/136 g
Yuzu

Essential Oil Alternative
4.5 ounces/128 g
lemongrass

Additives

6.5 ounces/184 g
sour cream
1 ounce/28 g
vitamin E oil

Colorants

Disperse each in 1 table-spoon/15 mL sweet almond oil.

1 teaspoon/5 ml
Yellow mica
1 teaspoon/5 mL
Kermit Green mica
1 teaspoon/5 mL
Racing Stripe Orange mica

Natural Colorant Alternative
3 teaspoons/15 mL
ultramarine pink pigment
1 teaspoon/5 mL
yellow oxide
1 teaspoon/5 mL
green oxide

Safe Soaping!

Wear proper safety gear the whole time · Work in a well-ventilated space · No distractions

Use Any Milk

As with all these recipes, you can substitute any other kind of milk or dairy product, used in the same amount.

Prepare Ahead

Make the sour cream if you are using homemade. Note that homemade sour cream may turn out thinner than a store-bought version. If you use a commercial brand, choose one with as few additives as possible.

Place the silicone liner in the mold. Assemble the dividers and keep them nearby.

Make the Soap Batter

1 Melt the palm oil in its original container, mix it thoroughly, and measure it into a heatproof bowl large enough to hold the entire recipe. Melt and measure the coconut oil and add it to the bowl. Add the shea butter to the hot oils and stir until melted. If needed, microwave the bowl in 10-second bursts to melt the butter completely. Add the avocado oil, hempseed oil, olive oil, sweet almond oil, and castor oil and set the bowl aside.

2 Measure the distilled water and the lye into separate heatproof containers. Add the lye to the water a tablespoon (15 mL) at a time (never add the liquid to the lye). Stir continuously until the lye fully dissolves and the water becomes clear. Stir the sodium lactate into the lye-water.

3 When the oils and the lye-water have cooled to about 105°F (40.5°C), add the lye-water to the oils, pouring it over the shaft of the stick blender to minimize air bubbles.

4 Insert the stick blender into the batter, tilting it so that any trapped air can escape. *Do not turn on the stick blender until the blades are fully immersed.* Alternate pulsing and stirring with the stick blender until you reach emulsion.

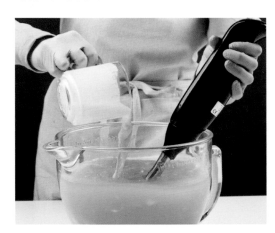

5 Add the fragrance oil, sour cream, and vitamin E. Stick-blend until combined and at thin trace.

Color the Soap

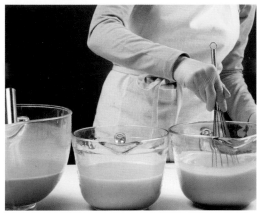

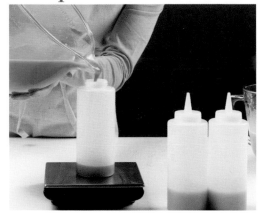

6 Split the batter evenly among the three bowls; there should be about 33 ounces (936 g) in each. Add one colorant to each bowl and stir by hand to combine.

7 Pour 3 ounces (85 g) of each color into its own squirt bottle, then cap the bottles and set them aside.

Pour and Swirl

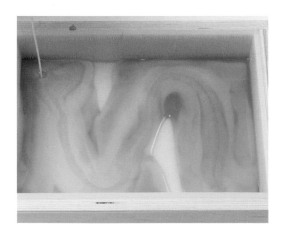

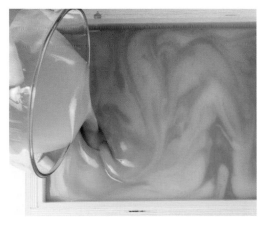

8 Pour thick horizontal zigzags of color into the mold from the bowls, alternating colors until all the batter in the bowls is used.

9 The colors will fill in and overlap as the layers are poured.

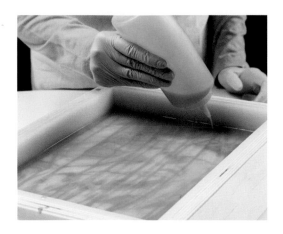

10 Squirt thin lines of color onto the batter across the length of the mold. (Shake the bottles first, if needed, to loosen the batter.)

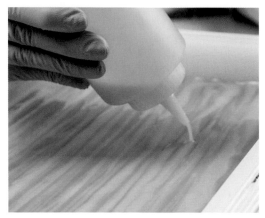

11 Alternate colors until all the batter is used, making sure the top and final layer has neat straight lines.

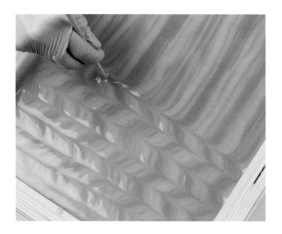

12 Insert the chopstick all the way to the bottom at one corner of the mold and drag it along the short side of the mold to the other corner. Move it about a ½ inch along the long side, then drag it across the soap to make a line. Repeat the pattern back and forth across the entire mold.

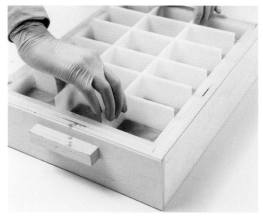

13 Insert the dividers.

Final Steps

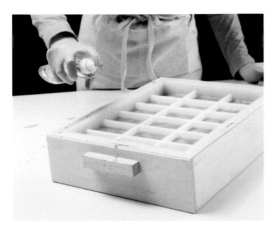

14 Spray thoroughly with 99% rubbing alcohol several times over 90 minutes to prevent soda ash. Let sit at least 48 hours at room temperature before unmolding. Optional: bevel the top edges of each bar to reveal even more of the design.

15 Let the bars cure in a well-ventilated area for 4 to 6 weeks before using, turning them every few days to ensure they cure evenly.

TECHNIQUE TIP

Use sliding or twisting motions to release the soaps from the dividers. Pulling the dividers directly away from the bars will tear the soaps and leave jagged sides.

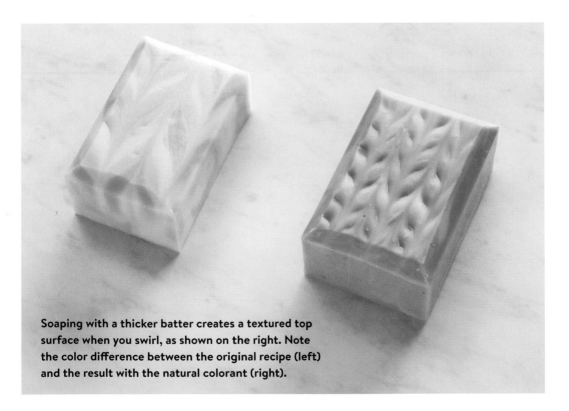

Soaping with a thicker batter creates a textured top surface when you swirl, as shown on the right. Note the color difference between the original recipe (left) and the result with the natural colorant (right).

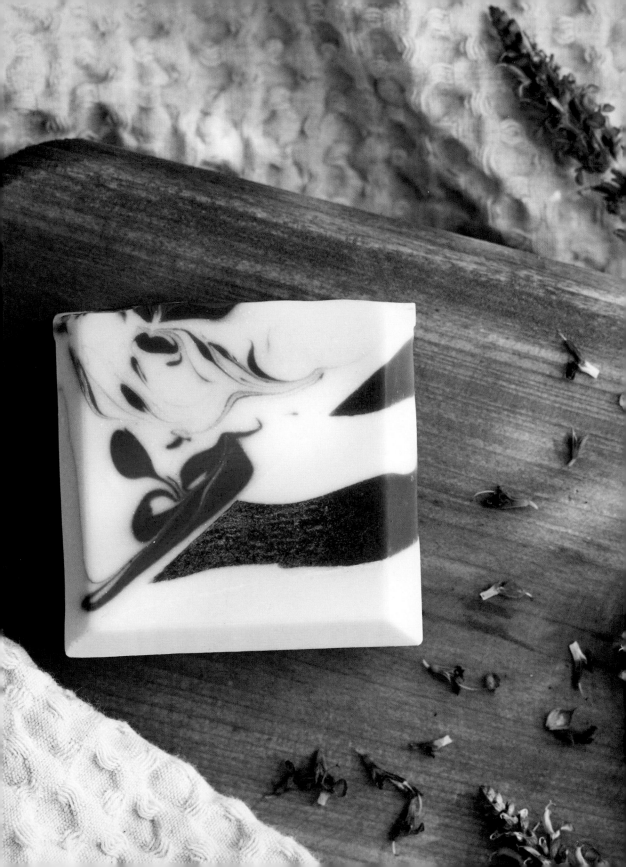

Floral Layers
Goat's Milk Bars

IOO% REPLACEMENT • MAKES I2 BARS

Goat's milk and avocado butter create a skin-loving, all-natural bar that is delicately colored with oxides and divinely scented with essential oils. The advanced floral design paired with stripes creates an optical illusion that makes people wonder, "How did they do that?!" We saw this design on Tania Vivian's YouTube channel, Soapish, and were inspired to make a version for this book.

This recipe requires two batches of soap and takes at least two days of soaping to complete.

STAGE 1: MAKE THE STRIPED SOAP

Mold and Special Tools
4-pound (1.8 kg)
  wood loaf mold
2 (2-pound/907 g)
  silicone liners
Fine-mesh strainer
4 easy-pour containers
Wire soap slicer

Oil Amounts
6.0 ounces/170 g
  coconut oil (30%)
6.0 ounces/170 g
  palm oil (30%)
5.0 ounces/142 g
  pure olive oil (25%)
2.0 ounces/57 g
  avocado butter (10%)

1.0 ounce/28 g
  castor oil (5%)

Lye Mixture
6.6 ounces/187 g
  goat's milk, frozen
2.9 ounces/82 g
  lye (3% superfat)
2 teaspoons/10 mL
  sodium lactate*

This recipe calls for slicing the loaf 24 hours after it has been poured. Sodium lactate, while normally optional, helps the loaf set fast enough for that to be possible, so we do not recommend leaving it out.

Essential Oil Blend
0.8 ounce/23 g
  lavender 40/42
0.5 ounce/14 g
  Egyptian geranium
0.3 ounce/8.5 g
  bergamot

Colorants
1 teaspoon/5 mL
  titanium dioxide dispersed
  into 1 tablespoon/15 mL
  olive oil
1 teaspoon/5 mL
  ultramarine violet oxide
  dispersed into 1 table-
  spoon/15 mL olive oil

Safe Soaping!
Wear proper safety gear the whole time · Work in a well-ventilated space · No distractions

Use Any Milk
As with all these recipes, you can substitute any other kind of milk or dairy product, used in the same amount.

Make the Striped Soap Batter

1 Melt the palm oil in its original container, mix it thoroughly, and measure it into a heatproof bowl large enough to hold the entire recipe. Melt and measure the coconut oil and add it to the bowl. Add the avocado butter to the hot oils and stir until melted. If needed, microwave the bowl in 10-second bursts to melt the butter completely. Add the olive oil and castor oil and set the bowl aside.

2 Measure the frozen milk and the lye into separate heatproof containers. Slowly add the lye to the milk a tablespoon (15 mL) at a time, stirring continuously until all the lye has fully dissolved. This can take up to 30 minutes due to the cold temperature.

Add the sodium lactate to the lye mixture and stir to combine.

3 When the oils have cooled to between 100 and 105°F (38–40.5°C) and the lye mixture is between 75 and 85°F (24–29°C), gently pour the lye mixture through the strainer into the oils, stirring any residue gently with a spatula.

4 Insert the stick blender into the batter, tilting it so that any trapped air can escape. *Do not turn on the stick blender until the blades are fully immersed.* Alternate pulsing and stirring with the stick blender until a medium trace is achieved.

Color the Soap

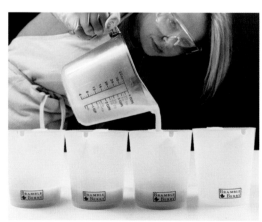

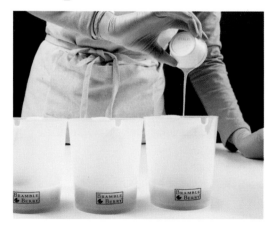

5 Divide the batter evenly into four easy-pour containers. You should have about 6 ounces (177 g) in each container.

6 Add 1 teaspoon (5 mL) of dispersed ultra-marine violet oxide to two containers. Add 1 teaspoon (5 mL) of dispersed titanium dioxide to the other two containers.

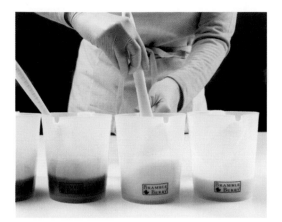

7 Divide the essential oil blend evenly among the four containers and mix in, pulsing with the stick blender for a few seconds if needed to blend well and help reach medium trace.

Pour the Soap

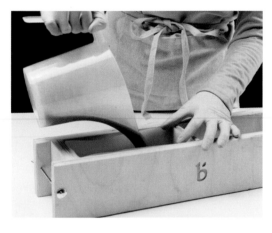

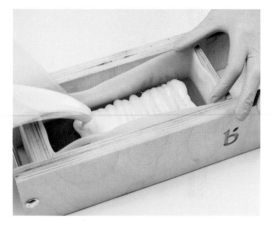

8 Pour one container of violet into the mold, using all the batter. Gently tap the mold on the counter to settle the soap and even out the top.

9 Pour one container of white batter on top of the violet, pouring low and slow so it doesn't break through. Tap the mold again.

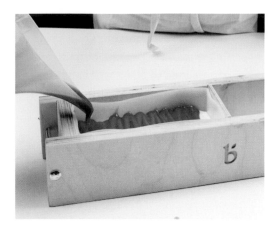

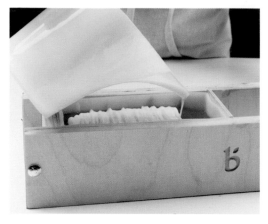

10 Pour the second container of violet. Again, use all the batter and layer it evenly over the white layer, being careful not to break through.

11 Pour the second container of white batter to create the final layer. Tap the mold again to settle to soap and even out the top.

Final Steps

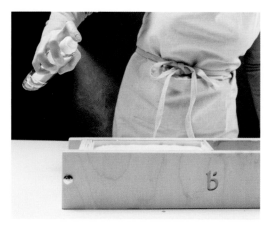

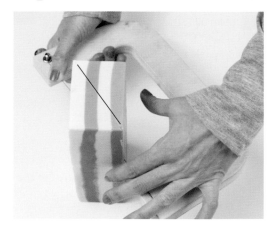

12 Spray thoroughly with 99% rubbing alcohol several times over 90 minutes to prevent soda ash. Let sit for 24 hours at room temperature before unmolding.

13 Unmold your soap and stand it on end. Slice the loaf diagonally from the top to bottom. Place both liners into the loaf mold and place a freshly cut half loaf into each side with the cut side up. Cover the mold with plastic wrap until you are ready to pour the second batch.

TECHNIQUE TIP

It can help to pour each layer slowly over the back of a spatula to keep the layers from breaking through.

STAGE 2: MAKE THE FLORAL SOAP

Mold and Special Tools

4-pound (1.8 kg)
   wood loaf mold
2 (2-pound/907 g)
   silicone liners
Fine-mesh strainer
3 easy-pour containers
Hanger swirl tool
   (see page 130)

Oil Amounts

7.2 ounces/204 g
   coconut oil (30%)
7.2 ounces/204 g
   palm oil (30%)
6.0 ounces/170 g
   pure olive oil (25%)

2.4 ounces/68 g
   avocado butter (10%)
1.2 ounces/34 g
   castor oil (5%)

Lye Mixture

7.9 ounces/224 g
   goat's milk, frozen
3.5 ounces/99 g
   lye (3% superfat)
2 teaspoons/10 mL
   sodium lactate*

Recommended to keep both loaves the same and prevent separation.

Essential Oil Blend

0.3 ounce/8.5 g
   bergamot

0.5 ounce/14 g
   Egyptian geranium
0.8 ounce/23 g
   lavender 40/42

Colorants

1 teaspoon/5 mL
   ultramarine pink oxide
   dispersed into 1 table-
   spoon/15 mL olive oil
1 teaspoon/5 mL
   green chrome oxide
   dispersed into 1 table-
   spoon/15 mL olive oil
2 teaspoons/10 mL
   titanium dioxide dispersed
   into 2 tablespoons/30 mL
   olive oil

Make the Floral Soap Batter

1 Melt the palm oil in its original container, mix it thoroughly, and measure it into a heatproof bowl large enough to hold the entire recipe. Melt and measure the coconut oil and add it to the bowl. Add the avocado butter to the hot oils and stir until melted. If needed, microwave the bowl in 10-second bursts to melt the butter completely. Add the olive oil and castor oil and set the bowl aside.

2 Measure the frozen milk and the lye into separate heatproof containers. Slowly add the lye to the milk a tablespoon (15 mL) at a time, stirring continuously until all the lye has fully dissolved. This can take up to 30 minutes due to the cold temperature. Add the sodium lactate to the lye mixture and stir to combine.

3 When the oils have cooled to between 100 and 105°F (38–40.5°C) and the lye mixture is between 75 and 85°F (24–29°C), gently pour the lye mixture through the strainer into the oils, stirring any residue gently with a spatula.

4 Insert the stick blender into the batter, tilting it so that any trapped air can escape. *Do not turn on the stick blender until the blades are fully immersed.* Alternate pulsing and stirring with the stick blender until a thin trace is achieved.

Color, Pour, and Swirl

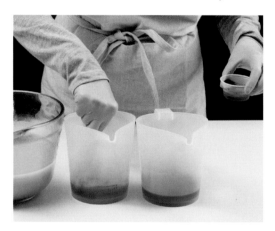 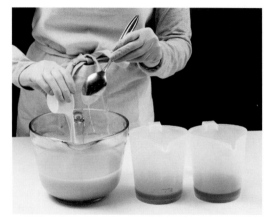

5 Pour 3 ounces (85 g) of soap batter into each easy-pour container. Add ½ teaspoon (2.5 mL) dispersed ultramarine pink oxide to one container and stir in by hand. Add ½ teaspoon (2.5 mL) dispersed green chrome oxide to the other and stir in by hand.

6 Mix all of the dispersed titanium dioxide into the remaining batter by hand.

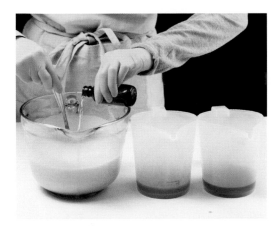

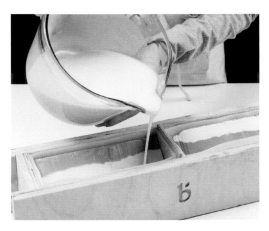

7 Add the essential oils to the white batter and stir in.

8 Pour the white batter into each mold until the bottom two layers of the first loaves are covered.

TECHNIQUE TIP

Transfer it to an easy pour container, refilling as needed, to make pouring and designing easier.

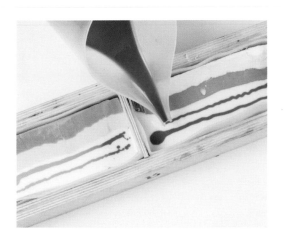

9 Pour two green lines down the length of each mold, close to each other and near the center of the newly poured batter. Pour from a little higher so the batter breaks through a bit. Save just a couple spoonfuls for the top design; you won't need much.

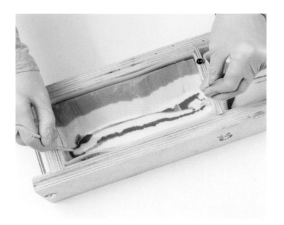

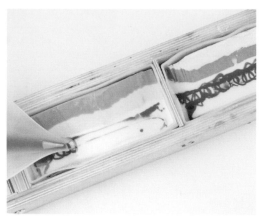

10 To create the stems and leaves, line up the hanger swirl tool along a green line. Push the tool straight to the bottom of the mold, slide it through the batter, then pull it straight up and out. Repeat on the second green line. Wipe off the tool and keep it handy.

11 To create the flowers, alternate pouring white and pink batter in a swirl design; try not to break through to the green.

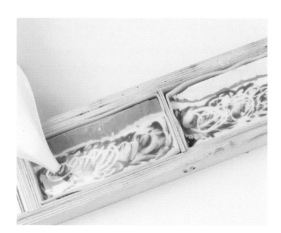

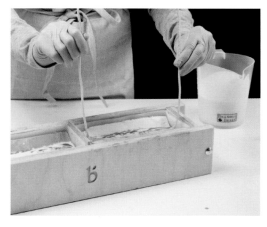

12 Save enough white batter for a final thin layer on top and save a couple spoonfuls of pink for a single line on top of each loaf.

13 Use the hanger swirl tool to create small loops through the pink and white batters, being careful not to break through to the green stems.

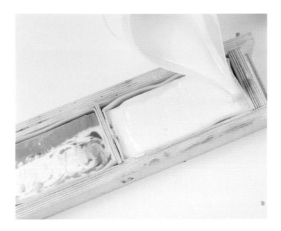

14 Cover the swirls with a thin layer of white soap batter. Too much batter will weigh down and flatten the design, so pour lightly.

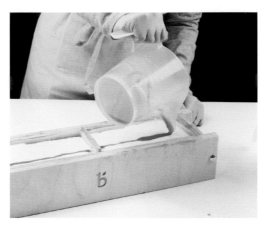

15 Pour a thin line of pink batter along the side of the mold with the freshly poured batter.

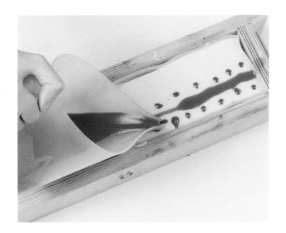

16 Add little green dots of batter along both sides of this line.

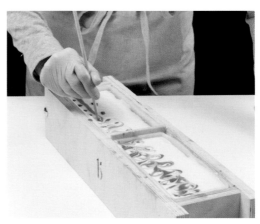

17 Gently insert a chopstick into the very top layer to swirl a pattern of infinity symbols through the lines and dots down the length of the mold.

Final Steps

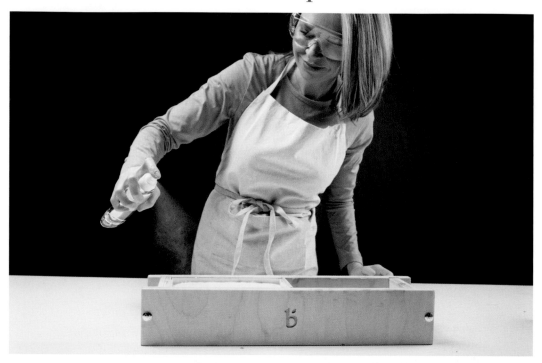

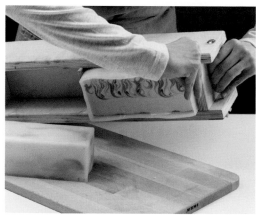

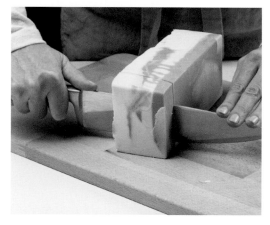

18 Spray thoroughly with 99% rubbing alcohol several times over 90 minutes to prevent soda ash. Let sit for at least 48 hours at room temperature before unmolding and slicing into bars.

19 Let the bars cure in a well-ventilated area for 4 to 6 weeks before using, turning them every few days to ensure they cure evenly.

Circling Taiwan Swirl
with Matcha Tea

100% REPLACEMENT • MAKES 8 BARS

This advanced recipe uses the stunning circling Taiwan swirl technique, made popular by Elaine Wright of Misty Springs Bath & Body in Royersford, Pennsylvania. It contains 10 percent matcha green tea butter and is infused with matcha tea powder for an antioxidant boost. The special final cut reveals the stunning design inside.

Mold and Special Tools

10-inch (25 cm) silicone loaf mold
Plastic mold dividers
Iron
Heat-sealable tea bag
Chopstick
4 easy-pour containers
Fine-mesh strainer
Soap beveller (optional)

Oil Amounts

9.9 ounces/281 g
    pure olive oil (30%)
6.6 ounces/187 g
    palm oil (20%)
4.9 ounces/139 g
    coconut oil (15%)
4.9 ounces/139 g
    sweet almond oil (15%),
    infused (see page 203)

3.3 ounces/94 g
    matcha green tea butter
    (10%)
1.6 ounces/45 g
    hempseed oil (5%)
1.6 ounces/45 g
    castor oil (5%)

Lye Mixture

10.8 ounces/306 g
    hazelnut milk, frozen
4.5 ounces/128 g
    lye (4% superfat)
3 teaspoons/15 mL
    sodium lactate

Essential Oil Blend

1.0 ounce/28 g
    patchouli
1.0 ounce/28 g
    lime
0.2 ounce/6 g
    spearmint

Colorants

Disperse each into 1 tablespoon (15 mL) sweet almond oil.

1 teaspoon/5 mL
    green iron oxide
1 teaspoon/5 mL
    titanium dioxide
1 teaspoon/5 mL
    brown oxide

Additives

1 ounce/28 g
    vitamin E oil
1 tablespoon/15 mL
    matcha green tea powder

Safe Soaping!

Wear proper safety gear the whole time · Work in a well-ventilated space · No distractions

Use Any Milk

As with all these recipes, you can substitute any other kind of milk or dairy product, used in the same amount.

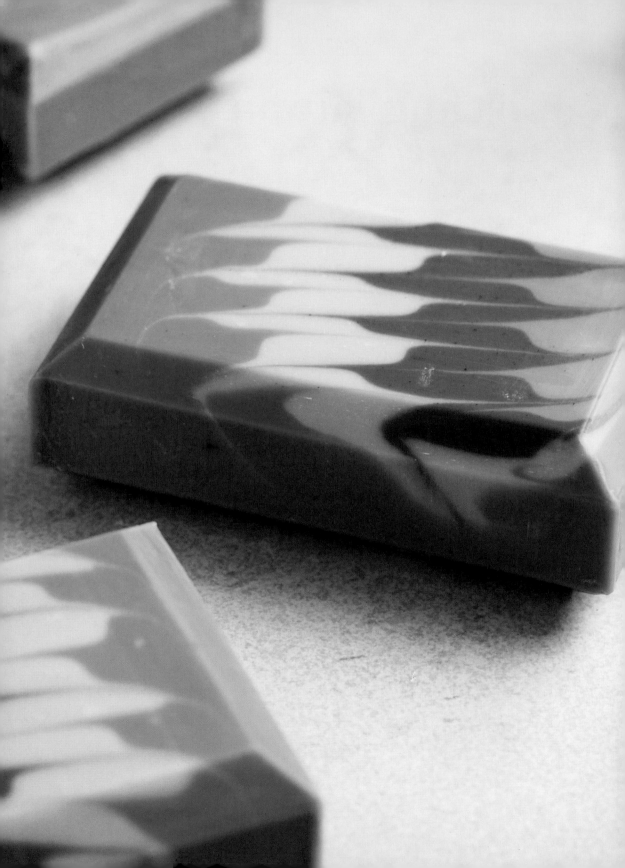

Prepare Ahead

1 Make the hazelnut milk according to the instructions on page 8; freeze.

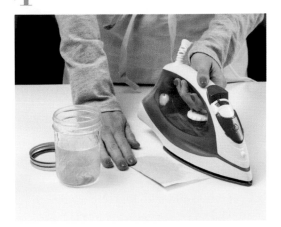

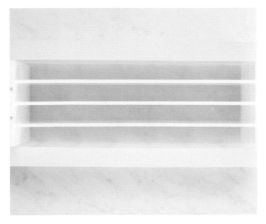

2 Place the matcha tea powder into the heat-sealable tea bag and seal with the iron. Place this into a container of 5.2 ounces (147 g) sweet almond oil. Let sit for at least 24 hours to infuse into the oil. (You want to infuse a little extra oil, as some will be absorbed.)

3 Set up the plastic dividers so that you have three long dividers and two end pieces, making four areas to pour batter into. Press the dividers firmly into the mold.

Make the Soap Batter

1 Melt the palm oil in its original container, mix it thoroughly, and measure it into a heatproof bowl large enough to hold the entire recipe. Melt and measure the coconut oil and add it to the bowl. Add the matcha green tea butter to the hot oils and stir until melted. If needed, microwave the bowl in 10-second bursts to melt the butter completely. Add the olive oil, infused sweet almond oil, hempseed oil, and castor oil and set the bowl aside.

2 Measure the frozen milk and the lye into separate heatproof containers. Slowly add the lye to the milk a tablespoon (15 mL) at a time, stirring continuously until all the lye has fully dissolved. This can take up to 30 minutes due to the cold temperature. Add the sodium lactate to the lye mixture and stir to combine.

3 When the oils have cooled to between 100 and 105°F (38–40.5°C) and the lye mixture is between 75 and 85°F (24–29°C), gently pour the lye mixture through the strainer into the oils, stirring any residue gently with a spatula.

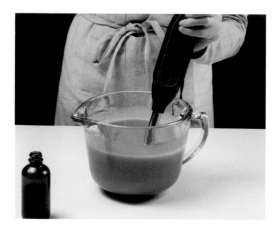

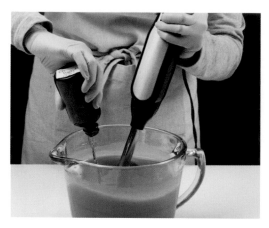

4 Insert the stick blender into the batter, tilting it so that any trapped air can escape. *Do not turn on the stick blender until the blades are fully immersed.* Alternate pulsing and stirring with the stick blender until you reach emulsion.

5 Add the essential oils and the vitamin E and stick-blend to thin trace.

Color and Pour

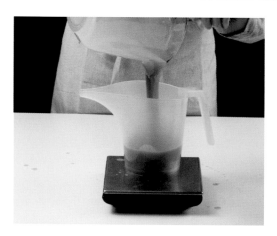

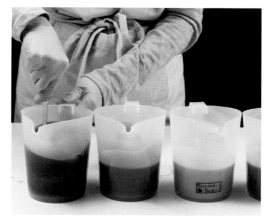

6 Divide the batter evenly into the four easy-pour containers, pouring about 12.5 ounces (354 g) into each.

7 Add ½ teaspoon (2.5 mL) brown oxide to one container, ½ teaspoon (2.5 mL) of green iron oxide to two containers, and 1 teaspoon (5 mL) of titanium to the fourth container, stirring each in by hand. You will have one brown batter, one white batter, and two green.

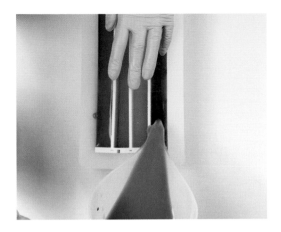

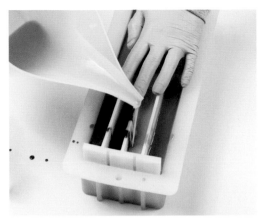

8 Holding the dividers in place with one hand, pour the two green batters into the outermost sections of the mold.

9 Still pressing the dividers down, pour the brown and the white batters into the center sections.

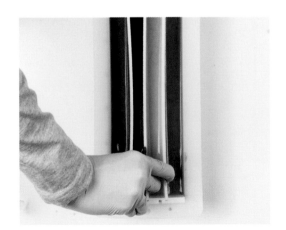

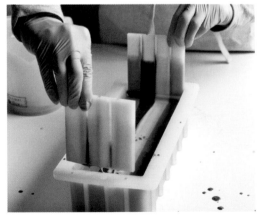

10 Carefully remove the dividers by pulling them straight up out of the mold.

Swirl

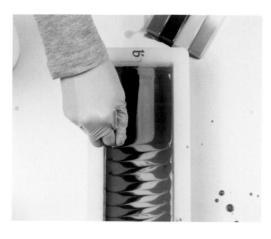 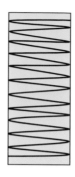

11 Insert the chopstick to the bottom of the mold, then swirl it side to side down the length of the mold. Keep the lines very tight and close together to improve the effect and appearance of the finished swirl.

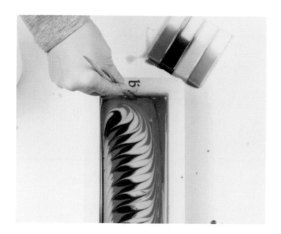 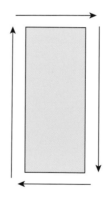

12 Now swirl the chopstick around the outer edges of the mold multiple times to pull the previously made lines into a circular pattern.

Final Steps

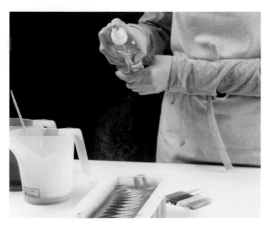

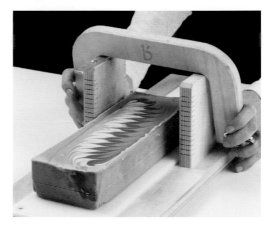

13 Spray thoroughly with 99% rubbing alcohol several times over 90 minutes to prevent soda ash. Let sit at room temperature for at least 48 hours before unmolding.

14 Remove the soap from the mold and slice lengthwise through the center to create two identical loaves.

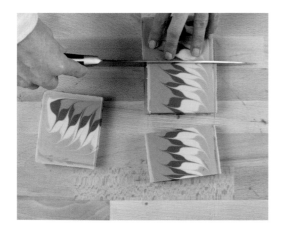

15 Slice each loaf into four bars. (This is the same technique used in the Super Rainbow Swirl [page 171] and Concentric Circle Swirls [page 221]. The only difference is that this recipe makes a single loaf.) Optional: bevel the edges of each bar to reveal even more of the design.

16 Let the bars cure in a well-ventilated area for 4 to 6 weeks before using, turning them every few days to ensure they cure evenly.

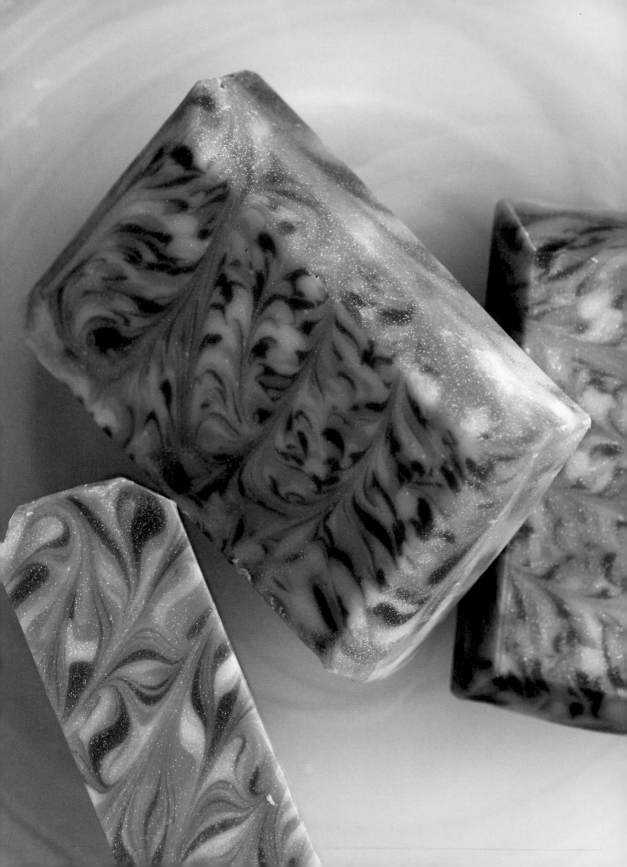

Squirty Swirls
with Whey

100% REPLACEMENT • MAKES 6 BARS

Did you know that you can use whey in place of milk to make soap? The soft oils in this recipe give you plenty of time to create a very moisturizing bar. The combination of squirt bottles and a hanger swirl tool lets you create fine, intricate swirls. The Snowflake Sparkle mica adds a delicate shimmer that can be hard to achieve in cold-process soap.

Mold and Special Tools

2-pound (907 g) wooden loaf mold
Fine-mesh strainer
Silicone liner for mold
4 easy-pour containers
4 squirt bottles
Hanger swirl tool (see page 130)
Soap beveller (optional)

Oil Amounts

6.6 ounces/187 g pure olive oil (30%)
4.4 ounces/125 g canola oil (20%)
4.4 ounces/125 g sweet almond oil (20%)
4.4 ounces/125 g coconut oil (20%)
1.1 ounces/31 g avocado oil (5%)
1.1 ounces/31 g castor oil (5%)

Lye Mixture

7.3 ounces/207 g whey, frozen
3.0 ounces/85 g lye (4% superfat)
2 teaspoons/10 mL sodium lactate

Fragrance Oil

1.6 ounces/45 g Crisp Cotton

Essential Oil Alternative
1.0 ounce/28 g lime
0.6 ounce/17 g Atlas cedarwood

Colorants

Disperse each combination into 1 tablespoon of canola oil.

¾ teaspoon (3.7 mL) Snowflake Sparkle + ¼ teaspoon (1.2 mL) Super Pearly White

¾ teaspoon (3.7 mL) Snowflake Sparkle + ¼ teaspoon (1.2 mL) Kelly Green

¾ teaspoon (3.7 mL) Snowflake Sparkle + ¼ teaspoon (1.2 mL) Luster Black

¾ teaspoon (3.7 mL) Snowflake Sparkle + ⅛ teaspoon (0.6 mL) Zippy Blue + ⅛ teaspoon (0.6 mL) Hydrated Chrome Green

Natural Colorant Alternative
Replace the mica colorants with titanium dioxide, green oxide, black oxide, and ultramarine blue pigment using ½ teaspoon (2.5 mL) of each dispersed colorant.

Safe Soaping!

Wear proper safety gear the whole time · Work in a well-ventilated space · No distractions

Use Any Milk

As with all these recipes, you can substitute any other kind of milk or dairy product, used in the same amount.

Make the Soap Batter

1 Melt and measure the coconut oil into a heatproof bowl large enough to hold the entire recipe. Add the canola oil, sweet almond oil, olive oil, avocado oil, and castor oil and set the bowl aside.

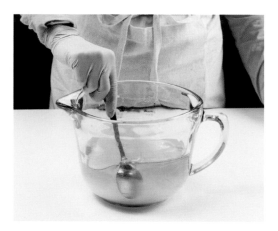

2 Measure the frozen whey and the lye into separate heatproof containers. Slowly add the lye to the whey a tablespoon (15 mL) at a time, stirring continuously until all the lye has fully dissolved. This can take up to 30 minutes due to the cold temperature. Add the sodium lactate to the lye mixture and stir to combine.

3 When the oils have cooled to between 100 and 105°F (38–40.5°C) and the lye mixture is between 75 and 85°F (24–29°C), gently pour the lye mixture through the strainer into the oils, stirring any residue gently with a spatula.

4 Insert the stick blender into the batter, tilting it so that any trapped air can escape. *Do not turn on the stick blender until the blades are fully immersed.* Alternate pulsing and stirring with the stick blender until a very thin trace is achieved.

Whey

Whey is a by-product of making cheese. It's best if you are able to use your own or obtain it from a cheese maker. Powdered whey is inferior because the manufacturing process strips the whey of its essential goodness: amino acids, vitamins, and probiotics.

You can also collect whey by draining two quarts of yogurt. (Don't use Greek yogurt, which has already been drained.) Set up a large colander lined with two layers of cheesecloth in a large bowl. Spoon the yogurt into the strainer and cover with a plate. Place the setup in the refrigerator for 6 to 8 hours (or overnight). Store the whey in the refrigerator for up to 5 days or freeze it in small amounts. The remaining thick yogurt can be flavored with salt and herbs and eaten like a spreadable cheese.

Color and Pour

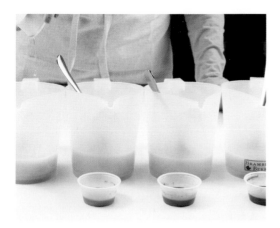

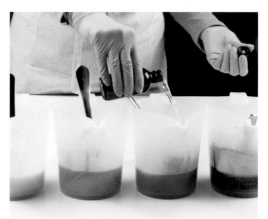

5 Divide the batter equally into four easy-pour containers (a little over 6.7 ounces/190 g in each). Add one dispersed colorant to each container. Stir well with a whisk or spoon.

6 Divide the fragrance equally among the four containers (it's okay to eyeball the amounts) and mix by hand. Do not stick-blend, as trace should be kept thin.

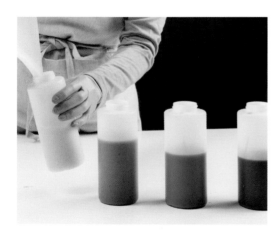

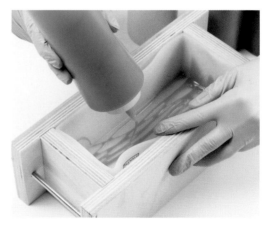

7 Pour each color into separate squirt bottles and put on the caps.

8 Make straight lines of soap batter down the length of the mold with one color, going down and back up the entire length of the mold several times.

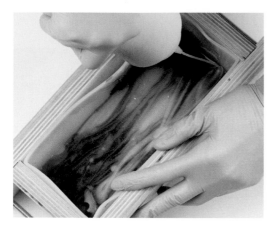

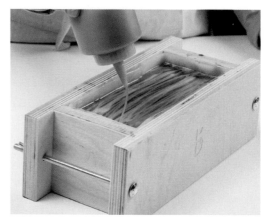

9 Repeat with the remaining colors, alternating them in order; for example, teal, black, green, white, repeat. Squirt the lines gently, close to the surface, so that they stack on top of one another rather than break through the other layers.

10 Continue until the mold is full, leaving a small amount of each color for the final design.

Make the Swirl

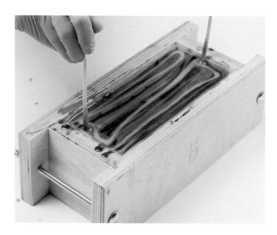

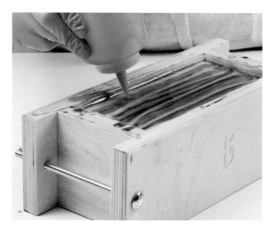

11 Moving the hanger swirl tool away from the side of the mold, make three or four large, overlapping circles without breaking the surface of the batter.

12 Squirt the remaining batter in straight lines across the top of the loaf.

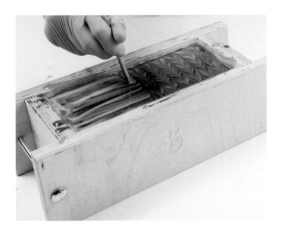

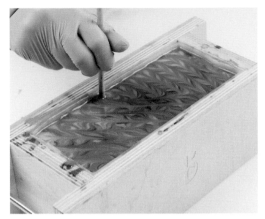

13 Gently insert a chopstick about ¼ inch into the soap at one corner of the mold. Make straight lines side to side across the width of the mold.

14 Starting in the same corner, insert the chopstick to the same depth and make straight diagonal lines to the opposite corner.

Final Steps

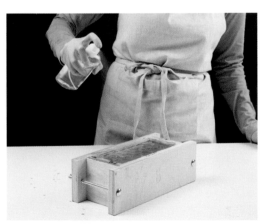

15 Spray thoroughly with 99% rubbing alcohol several times over 90 minutes to prevent soda ash. Let sit at room temperature for at least 48 hours before unmolding.

16 Slice into bars and bevel the edges of each bar if you wish.

17 Let the bars cure in a well-ventilated area for 4 to 6 weeks before using, turning them every few days to ensure they cure evenly.

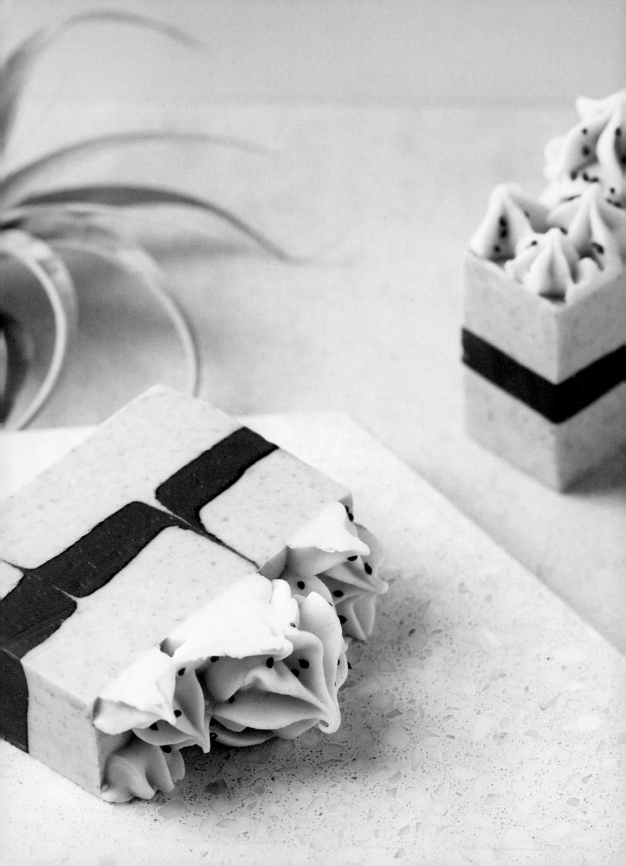

Piped Hanger Swirl
with Soy Milk

100% REPLACEMENT • MAKES 6 BARS

This striking design uses orange peel powder to provide both color and gentle exfoliation. With extra omega-3 from the soy milk plus 15 percent shea butter and 15 percent shea oil, this is a moisturizing and skin-loving bar. The top of the bar is textured with a frosting technique, adding to the interest of the design.

The hanger-swirl technique was inspired by Melanie Maddock of Sweet Escape Soap Company in New Zealand.

Mold and Special Tools

2-pound (907 g) wooden loaf mold with silicone liner
Powder duster
4 easy-pour containers
1M frosting tip
Disposable frosting bag
Hanger swirl tool (see page 130)
Fine-mesh strainer

Oil Amounts

4.4 ounces/125 g coconut oil (20%)
4.4 ounces/125 g palm oil (20%)
3.3 ounces/94 g shea butter (15%)
3.3 ounces/94 g shea oil (15%)
3.3 ounces/94 g sweet almond oil (15%)
2.2 ounces/62 g palm kernel flakes (10%)
1.1 ounces/31 g castor oil (5%)

Lye Mixture

7.26 ounces/206 g soy milk, frozen
3.0 ounces/85 g lye (7% superfat)
2 teaspoons/10 mL sodium lactate

Fragrance Oil

1.6 ounces/45 g red Brazilian mandarin essential oil

Colorants

1 teaspoon/5 mL Burgundy pigment dispersed into 1 tablespoon/15 mL sweet almond oil
1 teaspoon/5 mL titanium dioxide dispersed into 1 tablespoon/15 mL sweet almond oil
2–3 teaspoons/10–15 mL activated charcoal (for pencil lines; not dispersed)

Additives

2 teaspoons/10 mL orange peel powder
Approximately ¼ teaspoon/1.25 mL cranberry seeds

Safe Soaping!

Wear proper safety gear the whole time · Work in a well-ventilated space · No distractions

Use Any Milk

As with all these recipes, you can substitute any other kind of milk or dairy product, used in the same amount.

Prepare Ahead

Make the soy milk, using dry soybeans, according to the instructions on page 8; freeze. If you use commercial soy milk, choose an unflavored one with as few additives as possible.

Assemble your frosting bag by cutting off the tip and inserting the frosting tip.

Make the Soap Batter

1 Melt the palm oil in its original container, mix it thoroughly, and measure it into a heatproof bowl large enough to hold the entire recipe. Melt and measure the coconut oil and add it to the bowl. Add the shea butter and palm kernel flakes to the hot oils and stir until melted. If needed, microwave the bowl in 10-second bursts to melt the butter completely. Add the shea oil, sweet almond oil, and castor oil and set the bowl aside.

2 Measure the frozen milk and the lye into separate heatproof containers. Slowly add the lye to the milk a tablespoon (15 mL) at a time, stirring continuously until all the lye has fully dissolved. This can take up to 30 minutes due to the cold temperature. Add the sodium lactate to the lye mixture and stir to combine.

3 When the oils have cooled to between 100 and 105°F (38–40.5°C) and the lye mixture is between 75 and 85°F (24–29°C), gently pour the lye mixture through the strainer into the oils, stirring any residue gently with a spatula.

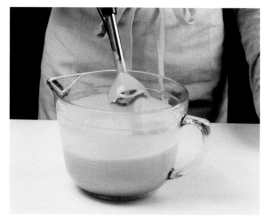

4 Insert the stick blender into the batter, tilting it so that any trapped air can escape. *Do not turn on the stick blender until the blades are fully immersed.* Alternate pulsing and stirring with the stick blender until a thin trace is achieved.

5 Stir in the essential oil.

Color and Pour

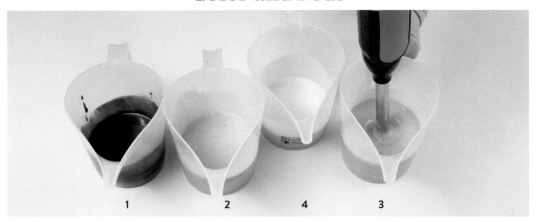

6 Pour the batter into the easy-pour containers and add the colorants as follows:
- Container 1: 6 ounces (170 g) batter + 1 teaspoon (5 mL) dispersed Burgundy pigment
- Container 2: 10 ounces (283 g) batter + 1 teaspoon (5 mL) orange peel powder
- Container 3: 10 ounces (283 g) batter + 1 teaspoon (5 mL) orange peel powder
- Container 4: 6 ounces (170 g) batter + 1 teaspoon (5 mL) dispersed titanium dioxide

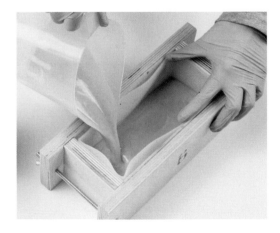

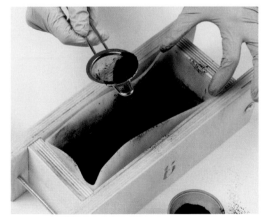

7 Stick-blend container 2 until the batter is thick enough to support layers but still pourable. Pour into the mold.

8 Top this layer with a thin pencil line: place 1–2 teaspoons (5–10 mL) of charcoal into the powder duster and gently tap over the soap to create a light dusting across the surface.

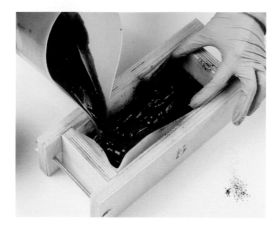

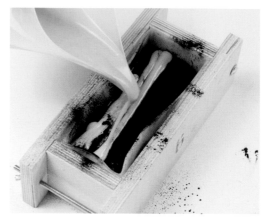

9 Stick-blend container 1 until the batter is thick enough to support layers but still pourable. Gently pour into the mold, layering on top of the charcoal without breaking through. Top with another thin charcoal pencil line.

10 Stick-blend container 3 until the batter is thick enough to support layers but still pourable. Pour this on top of the loaf, layering without breaking through.

Swirl and Pipe

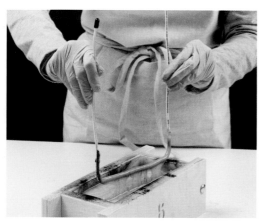

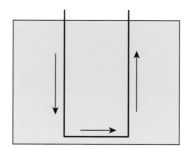

11 Insert the hanger swirl tool a third of the way in from one side of the mold, pushing it all the way to the bottom. Drag it one-third of the way toward the opposite side of the loaf, then pull it straight up and out.

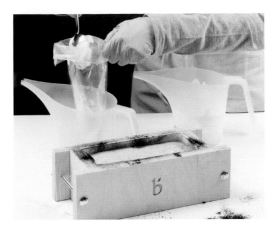

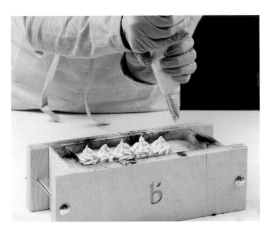

12 Stick-blend container 4 until the batter thickens. Let the batter sit for a few minutes to thicken even more, checking it with a spoon every couple of minutes. When you can make peaks in the batter that hold their shape, scoop the batter into the frosting bag.

13 Pipe a large row of dollops down the center of the loaf.

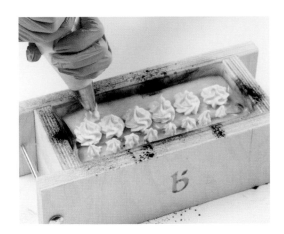

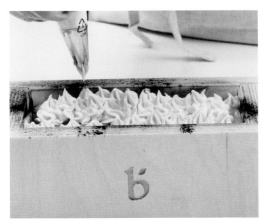

14 Pipe smaller dots along both sides, filling all the empty space.

15 Pipe a second row of large dollops on top of the first row to create a peak in the design.

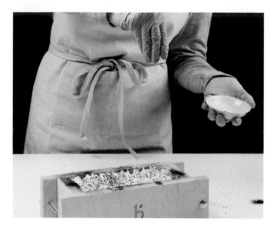

- It can help to pour each layer slowly over the back of a spatula to keep the layers from breaking through.

- Between layers, give each container a quick stir to keep the batters from setting up too much.

- If the charcoal lines are too thick, the layers can separate once the loaf is cut; keep them thin and even.

16 Sprinkle the cranberry seeds over the top of the loaf.

Final Steps

17 Spray thoroughly with 99% rubbing alcohol several times over 90 minutes to prevent soda ash. Set aside for 48 hours at room temperature before unmolding.

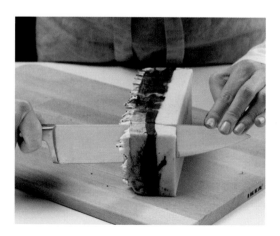

18 To cut the bars, lay the loaf on its side. This will protect the tops from damage, prevent the seeds from being dragged through the bars, and keep the pencil lines from smudging.

19 Let the bars cure in a well-ventilated area for 4 to 6 weeks before using, turning them every few days to ensure they cure evenly.

Concentric Circle Swirls
with Cashew Milk

100% REPLACEMENT • MAKES 16 BARS

This advanced technique uses slightly modified squirt bottle tops to create the large rings and a different cutting and beveling technique to make a whimsical design. But it's a slow-moving recipe, so you'll have plenty of time to make the concentric circles with the squirt bottles. A special cutting technique shows off this unusual design.

Mold and Special Tools

9-bar birchwood mold with silicone liner
4 squirt bottles with modified tops (see page 223)
Fine-mesh strainer
4 easy-pour containers
Wire soap slicer
Soap beveller (optional)

Oil Amounts

23.1 ounces/655 g
    pure olive oil (35%)
16.5 ounces/468 g
    sweet almond oil (25%)
9.9 ounces/281 g
    palm oil (15%)
9.9 ounces/281 g
    coconut oil (15%)
3.3 ounces/94 g
    mango butter (5%)
3.3 ounces/94 g
    castor oil (5%)

Lye Mixture

21.7 ounces/615 g
    cashew milk, frozen
8.9 ounces/252 g
    lye (5% superfat)
2 tablespoons/30 mL
    sodium lactate

Fragrance Oil

4.8 ounces/136 g
    Crisp Apple Rose

Essential Oil Alternative
3.2 ounces/91 g
    lemon
1.6 ounces/45 g
    peppermint
    2nd distilled

Colorants

Disperse the first two into 1 tablespoon/15 mL sweet almond oil.

1 teaspoon/5 mL
    Magenta mica
1 teaspoon/5 mL
    Evergreen mica
1 teaspoon/5 mL
    Gold Sparkle mica
2 teaspoons/10 mL
    titanium dioxide
    dispersed into 2 table-
    spoons/30 mL sweet
    almond oil

Natural Colorant Alternative
Replace the mica colorants with ultramarine pink pigment, green oxide, and yellow oxide at the same usage rates.

Safe Soaping!

Wear proper safety gear the whole time · Work in a well-ventilated space · No distractions

Use Any Milk

As with all these recipes, you can substitute any other kind of milk or dairy product, used in the same amount.

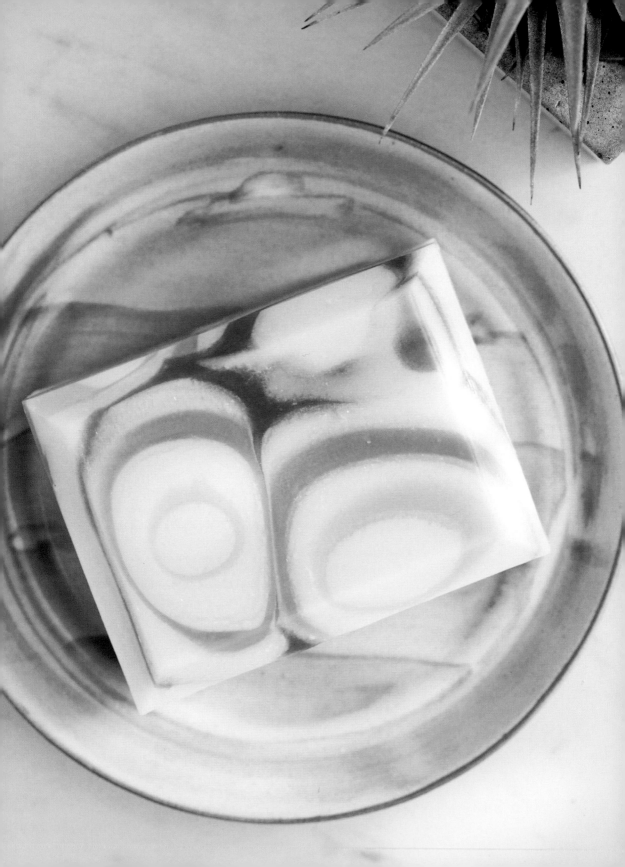

Prepare Ahead

Make the cashew milk according to the instructions on page 8; freeze.

Make the openings on the squirt bottle tops larger. If there are markings, cut down to the first line. If not, cut about ⅛ inch down.

Make the Soap Batter

1 Melt the palm oil in its original container, mix it thoroughly, and measure it into a heatproof bowl large enough to hold the entire recipe. Melt and measure the coconut oil and add it to the bowl. Add the mango butter to the hot oils and stir until melted. If needed, microwave the bowl in 10-second bursts to melt the butter completely. Add the castor oil, olive oil, and sweet almond oil and set the bowl aside.

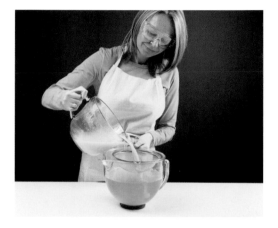

2 Measure the frozen milk and the lye into separate heatproof containers. Slowly add the lye to the milk a tablespoon (15 mL) at a time, stirring continuously until all the lye has fully dissolved. This can take up to 30 minutes due to the cold temperature. Add the sodium lactate to the lye mixture and stir to combine.

3 When the oils have cooled to between 100 and 105°F (38–40.5°C) and the lye mixture is between 75 and 85°F (24–29°C), gently pour the lye mixture through the strainer into the oils, stirring any residue gently with a spatula.

4 Insert the stick blender into the batter, tilting it so that any trapped air can escape. *Do not turn on the stick blender until the blades are fully immersed.* Alternate pulsing and stirring with the stick blender until a thin trace is achieved.

Color the Soap

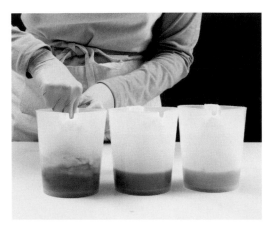

5 Pour about 7 ounces (198 g) of batter into three of the easy-pour containers. Add ½ teaspoon (2.5 mL) of dispersed mica, one color per container. Mix well by hand.

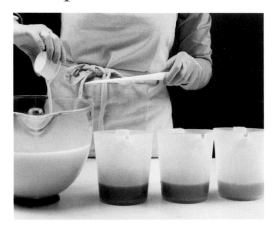

6 Add all of the dispersed titanium dioxide to the rest of the batter and stir in by hand.

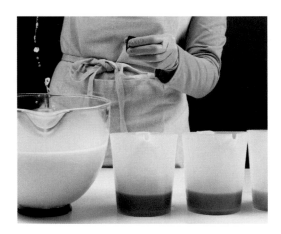

7 Add most of the fragrance to the large container of white batter, giving your colored batters a little bit as well; stir in by hand.

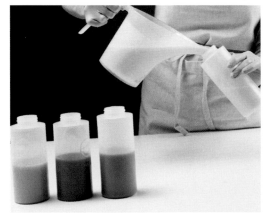

8 Pour the batters into the squirt bottles so you have one squirt bottle for each color, including white. Pour the white batter into the fourth easy-pour container to make it easier to fill the bottle. (The white will not all fit into the bottle, so you'll need to refill it.)

Pour the Soap

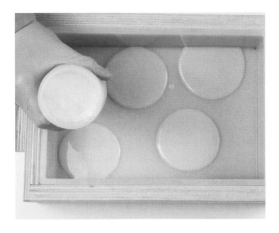

9 Squirt 4 or 5 white dots into the bottom of the mold.

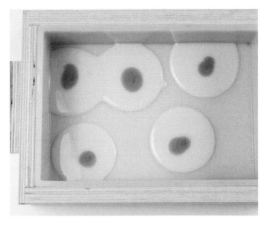

10 Squirt a smaller dot of another color directly in the middle of each white dot.

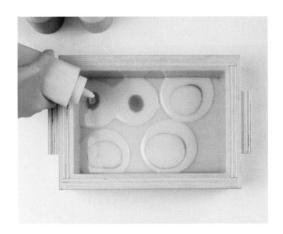

11 Make another series of white dots. The colored portion (the second squirt) will now look like a ring.

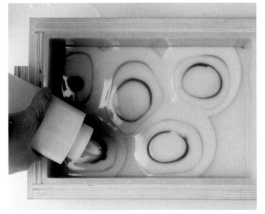

12 Continue with this pattern. Alternate colors, being heavy-handed with white. White should be squirted first, in between, and last.

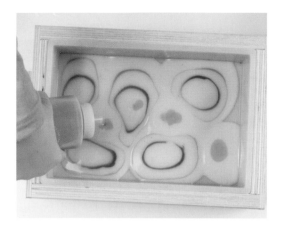
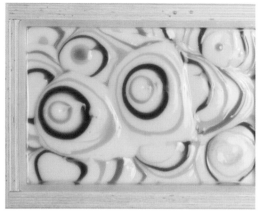

13 Start new circles on top of and between previous circles and continue until you fill the mold. Do not keep squirting into the same circles that you started with. This will distort some of the shapes; that is okay. **Note:** The bottles become slippery with drips of batter from the up-and-down motion of the pours, so handle them carefully.

Final Steps

14 Spray thoroughly with 99% rubbing alcohol several times over 90 minutes to prevent soda ash. Let sit at room temperature for at least 48 hours before unmolding.

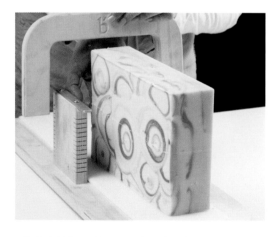
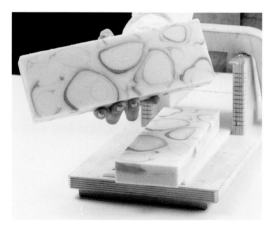

15 When the soap has hardened, remove it from the liner and cut lengthwise to make two rectangular loaves.

16 Slice each loaf lengthwise through the center, revealing the swirls inside.

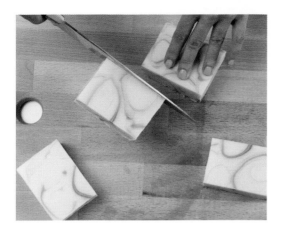

17 Cut each loaf into four individual bars. Bevel the top edges of each bar (four sides per bar) to reveal even more of the circle pattern.

18 Let the bars cure in a well-ventilated area for 4 to 6 weeks before using, turning them every few days to ensure they cure evenly.

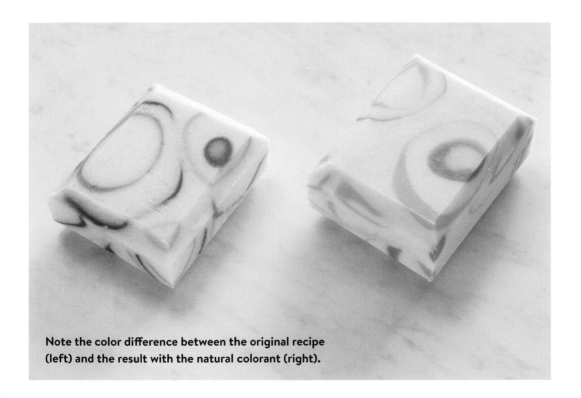

Note the color difference between the original recipe (left) and the result with the natural colorant (right).

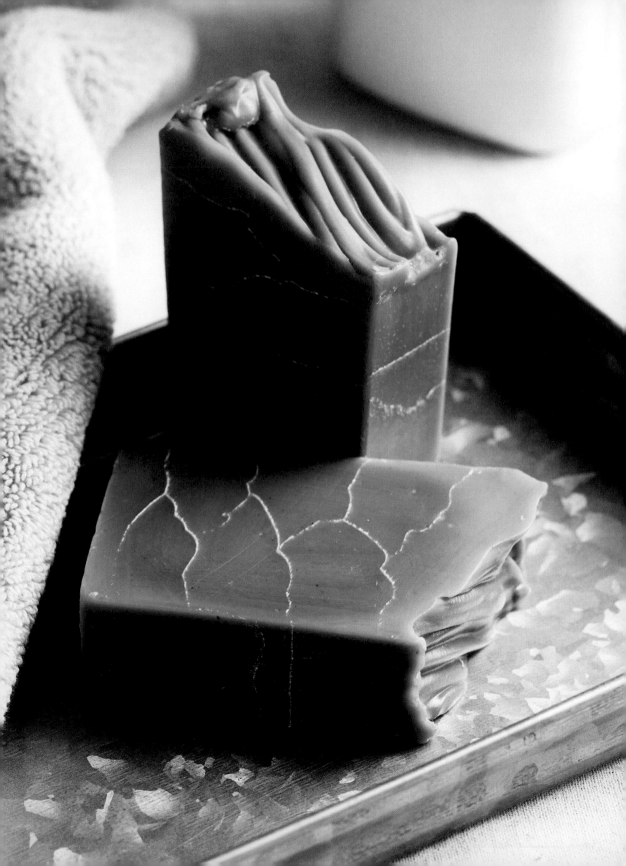

Alternating Layers
and Pencil Lines
with Flax Milk

30% ADDED AT TRACE • MAKES 10 BARS

This gorgeous design takes advantage of the natural tendencies of flax milk to accelerate the soap batter. You'll need to work quickly to create sloping layers and the white lines that stand out against the blue batter. A forked top texture creates even more visual interest, and mallow extract adds to the naturally soothing nature of this bar.

Note that the bars go in the freezer overnight to prevent overheating.

Mold and Special Tools

Tall 12-inch (30.5 cm) silicone loaf mold
Powder duster
Chopstick or pencil for propping up mold
Fork
Easy-pour container

Oil Amounts

8.5 ounces/241 g coconut oil (25%)
8.5 ounces/241 g palm oil (25%)
8.5 ounces/241 g apricot kernel oil (25%)
5.1 ounces/145 g rice bran oil (15%)
1.7 ounces/48 g shea butter (5%)
1.7 ounces/48 g castor oil (5%)

Lye-Water

7.8 ounces/221 g distilled water
4.6 ounces/130 g lye (7% superfat)
1 tablespoon/15 mL sodium lactate

Fragrance Oil

2.4 ounces/68 g Bramble Berry's Alien Type

Essential Oil Alternative
2.0 ounces/57 g lavender

Color

1 teaspoon/5 mL ultramarine blue pigment dispersed into 1 tablespoon/15 mL apricot kernel oil
2 tablespoons/30 mL titanium dioxide

Additives

3.3 ounces/94 g flax milk
1.5 ounces/43 g mallow extract

Safe Soaping!

Wear proper safety gear the whole time · Work in a well-ventilated space · No distractions

Use Any Milk

As with all these recipes, you can substitute any other kind of milk or dairy product, used in the same amount.

Prepare Ahead

Make the flax milk according to the instructions on page 10.

Grind the titanium dioxide in a coffee grinder for 30 to 45 seconds or until the powder is very fine. Be careful opening the grinder and transferring the titanium dioxide, as it can puff out all over the place.

Make the Soap Batter

1 Melt the palm oil in its original container, mix it thoroughly, and measure it into a heatproof bowl large enough to hold the entire recipe. Melt and measure the coconut oil and add it to the bowl. Add the shea butter to the hot oils and stir until melted. If needed, microwave the bowl in 10-second bursts to melt the butter completely. Add the rice bran oil, apricot kernel oil, and castor oil and set the bowl aside.

2 Measure the distilled water and the lye into separate heatproof containers. Add the lye to the water a tablespoon (15 mL) at a time (never add the liquid to the lye). Stir continuously until the lye fully dissolves and the water becomes clear. Stir the sodium lactate into the lye-water.

3 When the oils and the lye-water have cooled to about 105°F (40.5°C), add the lye-water to the oils, pouring it over the shaft of the stick blender to minimize air bubbles.

4 Insert the stick blender into the batter, tilting it so that any trapped air can escape. *Do not turn on the stick blender until the blades are fully immersed.* Alternate pulsing and stirring with the stick blender until a very thin trace is achieved.

Mix and Pour

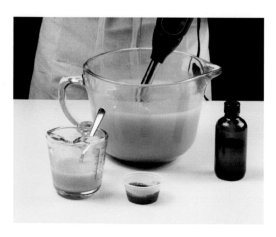

5 Add the mallow extract, fragrance oil, flax milk, and all of the dispersed blue colorant. The batter will thicken quickly, so don't overblend.

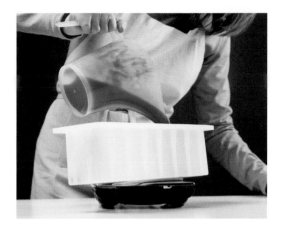

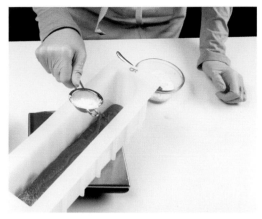

6 Pour some of the batter into the easy-pour container (you'll need to refill it). Place the mold on a scale and prop it at an angle by laying a chopstick under one of the long sides. Pour 5½ to 6 ounces (156–170 g) of batter along the lower side of the mold.

7 Place 1 teaspoon (5 mL) of titanium dioxide into the powder duster and gently tap it over of the blue soap to create a light dusting across the surface.

TECHNIQUE TIP

If the pencil lines are too thick, the layers can separate once the loaf is cut, so keep them thin and even.

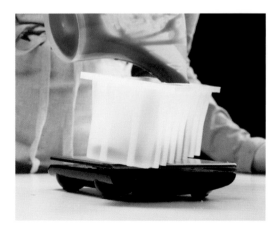

8 Move the chopstick to the other side so that the mold tilts the other way. Pour low and slow over the powder to create another layer.

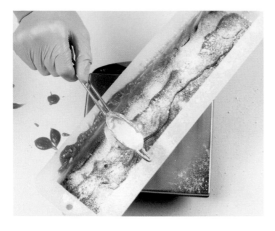

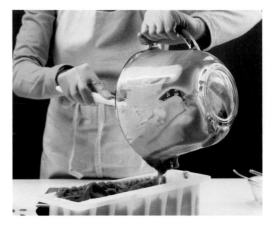

9 Continue alternating layers of batter and titanium dioxide, tilting the mold after every pour. You should have about seven layers and seven pencil lines, with enough batter left to make a final layer on top.

10 Lay the mold flat and pour or spoon the remaining batter on top. (It will continue to thicken as you pour, so you may need to scrape the bowl to create the last couple of layers.)

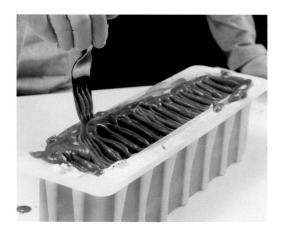

11 Use a fork to texture the top. We used the fork to pull batter up toward one longer side of the mold. Wipe the fork periodically with a paper towel to keep the tines from getting clogged with batter. Be careful not to disrupt the top pencil line by sticking the fork too far into the batter.

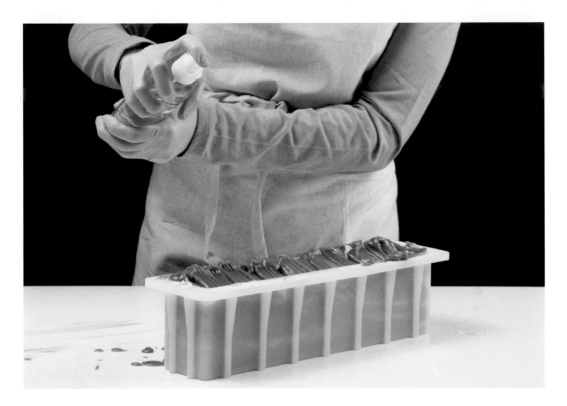

Final Steps

12 Spray thoroughly with 99% rubbing alcohol to prevent soda ash. To avoid a partial gel, either put the mold in the freezer or cover with a light blanket. The soaps shown here were covered and went through gel. If you don't gel, the blue will be slightly lighter.

13 Remove from the freezer and wait at least 48 hours before unmolding and cutting into bars. Frozen soaps tend to soften quite a bit as they thaw and need time to harden again.

14 Let the bars cure in a well-ventilated area for 4 to 6 weeks before using, turning them every few days to ensure they cure evenly.

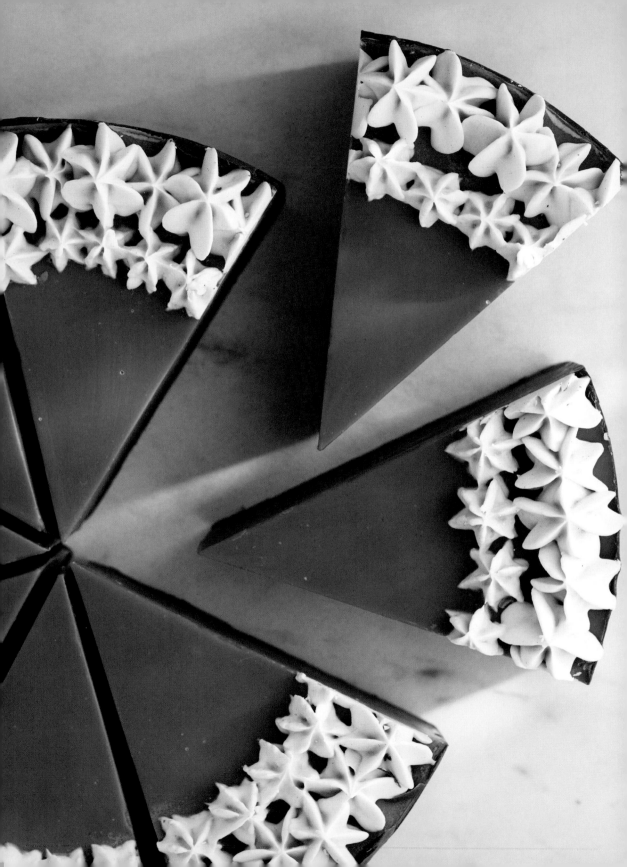

Double-Pumpkin
Pie Slices

I OO% REPLACEMENT • MAKES 8 "SLICES"

This classic pie soap uses a silicone cake-pan mold and piped soap frosting to make realistic-looking slices of pumpkin pie soap. Ground pumpkin seeds in the crust provide exfoliation. This recipe uses pumpkin seed milk for an extra-authentic pumpkin soap bar.

Mold and Special Tools

Silicone cake pan
Fine-mesh strainer
Disposable frosting bag
1M frosting tip
Extra stick-blending heads
 (optional; to thicken
 batters without mixing
 the colors)
4 easy-pour containers

Oil Amounts

12.3 ounces/349 g
 coconut oil (30%)
12.3 ounces/349 g
 palm oil (30%)
4.1 ounces/116 g
 cocoa butter (10%)
4.1 ounces/116 g
 palm kernel flakes (10%)
4.1 ounces/116 g
 shea butter (10%)

2.0 ounces/57 g
 pumpkin seed oil (5%)
2.0 ounces/57 g
 castor oil (5%)

Lye Mixture

13.5 ounces/383 g
 pumpkin seed milk,
 frozen
5.9 ounces/167 g
 lye (6% superfat)
3 teaspoons/15 mL
 sodium lactate

Fragrance Oil

2.4 ounces/68 g
 Pumpkin and Brown Sugar

Essential Oil Alternative
2 ounces/57 g
 orange 10x
0.4 ounce/11 g
 cinnamon

Colorants

Disperse the first two into
1 tablespoon/15 mL pumpkin
seed oil each.

1 teaspoon/5 mL
 brown oxide
1 teaspoon/5 mL
 Sunset Orange mica
2 teaspoons/10 mL
 titanium dioxide dispersed
 into 2 tablespoons/30 mL
 pumpkin seed oil

Natural Colorant Alternative
Replace the orange mica
with a dispersed mixture
of ¾ teaspoon/3.7 mL
yellow oxide and a scant
⅛ teaspoon/0.7 mL brick red
oxide; use entire dispersion.

Additive

2 teaspoons/10 mL
 ground pumpkin seeds

Safe Soaping!

Wear proper safety gear the whole time · Work in a well-ventilated space · No distractions

Use Any Milk

As with all these recipes, you can substitute any other kind of milk or dairy product,
used in the same amount.

Prepare Ahead

Make the pumpkin seed milk according to the instructions on page 8; freeze.

Assemble your frosting bag by cutting off the tip and inserting the frosting tip.

Make the Soap Batter

1 Melt the palm oil in its original container, mix it thoroughly, and measure it into a heatproof bowl large enough to hold the entire recipe. Melt and measure the coconut oil and add it to the bowl. Add the cocoa butter, palm kernel flakes, and shea butter to the hot oils and stir until melted. If needed, microwave the bowl in 10-second bursts to melt the butter completely. Add the pumpkin seed oil and castor oil and set the bowl aside.

2 Measure the frozen milk and the lye into separate heatproof containers. Slowly add the lye to the milk a tablespoon (15 mL) at a time, stirring continuously until all the lye has fully dissolved. This can take up to 30 minutes due to the cold temperature. Add the sodium lactate to the lye mixture and stir to combine.

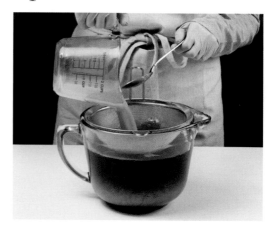

3 When the oils have cooled to between 100 and 105°F (38–40.5°C) and the lye mixture is between 75 and 85°F (24–29°C), gently pour the lye mixture through the strainer into the oils, stirring any residue gently with a spatula.

4 Insert the stick blender into the batter, tilting it so that any trapped air can escape. *Do not turn on the stick blender until the blades are fully immersed.* Alternate pulsing and stirring with the stick blender until a thin trace is achieved.

Color and Pour

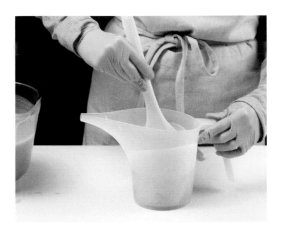

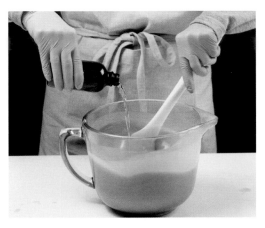

5 Pour 11.5 ounces (326 g) of batter into an easy-pour container and add all of the dispersed titanium dioxide. Mix well and set aside to thicken.

6 Stir the fragrance oil into the remaining batter by hand.

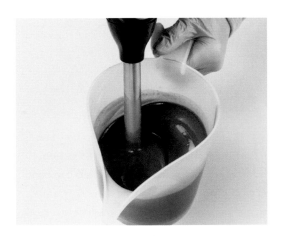

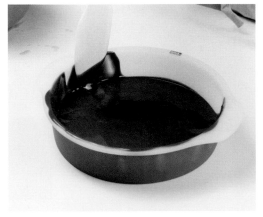

7 Pour 11.5 ounces (326 g) of the scented batter into an easy-pour container and add 1 teaspoon (5 mL) dispersed brown oxide and 2 teaspoons (10 mL) ground pumpkin seeds. Stick-blend until a medium/thick trace is achieved.

8 Pour the thickened brown batter into the cake pan. Use a spatula to spread the batter evenly around the bottom of the mold and up the sides to create the crust. Keep spreading batter up the sides until there is a thin layer up to the top.

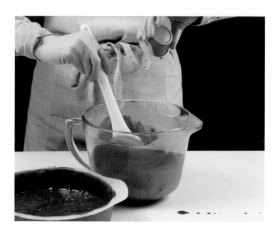

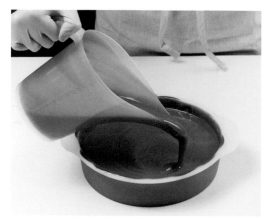

9 Add all of the dispersed Sunset Orange mica to the remainder of your original batter and transfer into an easy-pour container to make pouring the layers easier. Stick-blend if needed to thicken to medium trace.

10 Gently pour the orange batter into the mold to create the pie filling. Pour low and slow, layering the orange batter on top of the brown without breaking through.

TECHNIQUE TIP

It can help to pour each layer slowly over the back of a spatula to keep the layers from breaking through.

Pipe the Soap

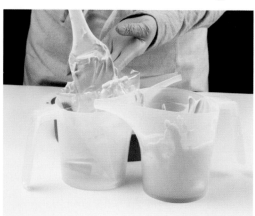

11 The white batter needs to be thick enough to pipe on top as frosting. Stick blend to thicken (this is where a second stick blender head comes in handy), then let sit to thicken further. Once it will hold a peak, scoop it into the frosting bag with a spatula. Use the extra easy-pour container to hold the frosting bag as you fill it.

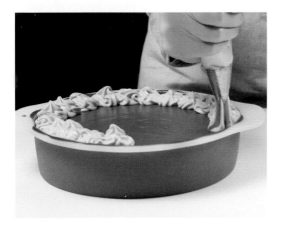

12 Pipe a ring of large dollops around the outer edge of the mold.

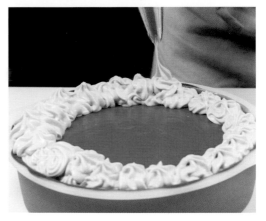

13 Pipe a second ring of dollops between the first dollops so that the entire outer edge is covered.

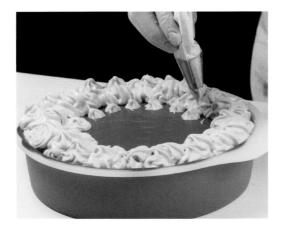

14 Pipe a row of smaller dollops in front of the bigger ones.

Final Steps

Spray thoroughly with 99% rubbing alcohol several times over 90 minutes to prevent soda ash. Let sit at least 48 hours at room temperature before unmolding.

Slice as you would a pie, into eight wedges. Let cure in a well-ventilated area for 4 to 6 weeks before using, turning the slices every few days to ensure they cure evenly. **Note:** The pie slices will darken as they cure.

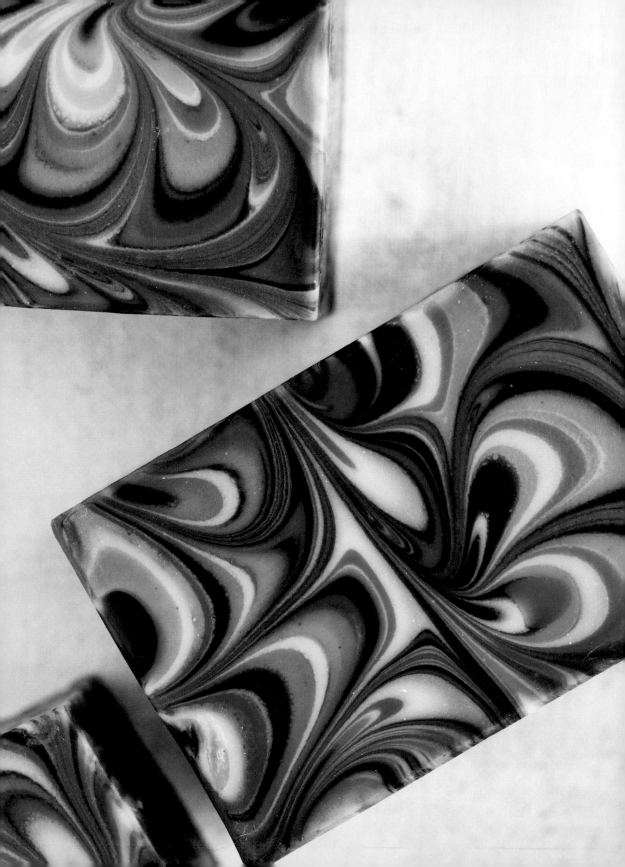

Elegant Swirls
with Hemp Milk and Avocado Extract

5 0 % added at trace • Makes 18 bars

This textured swirl technique uses a very thick trace and two different swirl tools to create the intriguing design. It's a bit tricky, so you need to work quickly to get it right. In addition to 8 percent avocado butter, this skin-loving bar includes fresh hemp milk and avocado extract for an extra-luxurious feel.

Mold and Special Tools

18-bar birchwood mold
Silicone liner and dividers
5 easy-pour containers
5 squirt bottles
Easy swirling tool
Comb swirling tool
Chopstick

Oil Amounts

19.8 ounces/561 g
   canola oil (30%)
15.8 ounces/448 g
   rice bran oil (24%)
13.2 ounces/374 g
   hempseed oil (20%)
6.6 ounces/187 g
   coconut oil (10%)
5.2 ounces/147 g
   avocado butter (8%)
3.3 ounces/94 g
   borage oil (5%)

1.9 ounces/54 g
   castor oil (3%)

Lye-Water

10.8 ounces/306 g
   distilled water
8.4 ounces/238 g
   lye (7% superfat)
2 tablespoons/30 mL
   sodium lactate

Fragrance Oil

4.7 ounces/136 g
   Fruity Fusion

Essential Oil Alternative

1.9 ounces/54 g
   Valencia orange
0.5 ounce/14 g
   Egyptian geranium

Colorants

Disperse each into 1 tablespoon/15 mL rice bran oil.

1 teaspoon/5 mL
   titanium dioxide
1 teaspoon/5 mL
   black oxide
1 teaspoon/5 mL
   Caribbean Blue mica
1 teaspoon/5 mL
   Raspberry mica
1 teaspoon/5 mL
   Queen's Purple mica

Natural Colorant Alternative

Replace the blue, raspberry, and purple colorants with ultramarine blue pigment, ultramarine pink pigment, and ultramarine violet pigment at the same usage rates.

Additives

10.8 ounces/306 g
   hemp milk
1.5 ounces/43 g
   avocado extract

Safe Soaping!

Wear proper safety gear the whole time · Work in a well-ventilated space · No distractions

Use Any Milk

As with all these recipes, you can substitute any other kind of milk or dairy product, used in the same amount.

Prepare Ahead

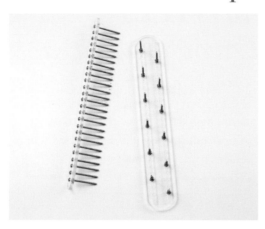

Make the hemp milk according to the instructions on page 8.

Assemble the swirling tools. The comb swirling tool should have all the screws in place. The easy swirling tool should have only every fourth screw inserted in an alternating pattern on the top and bottom rows, as shown.

Place the silicone liner into the mold. Assemble the dividers, but don't put them into the mold yet.

Make the Soap Batter

1 Melt and measure the coconut oil into a heatproof bowl large enough to hold the entire recipe. Add the avocado butter to the hot coconut oil and stir until melted. If needed, microwave the bowl in 10-second bursts to melt the butter completely. Add the borage oil, canola oil, hempseed oil, rice bran oil, and castor oil and set the bowl aside.

2 Measure the distilled water and the lye into separate heatproof containers. Add the lye to the water a tablespoon (15 mL) at a time (never add the liquid to the lye). Stir continuously until the lye fully dissolves and the water becomes clear. Stir the sodium lactate into the lye-water.

3 When the oils and the lye-water have cooled to about 105°F (40.5°C), add the lye-water to the oils, pouring it over the shaft of the stick blender to minimize air bubbles.

4 Insert the stick blender into the batter, tilting it so that any trapped air can escape. *Do not turn on the stick blender until the blades are fully immersed.* Alternate pulsing and stirring with the stick blender until a very thin trace is achieved.

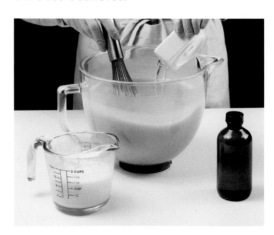

5 Add the avocado extract, fragrance oil, and hemp milk and whisk until blended, keeping trace thin.

Color and Pour

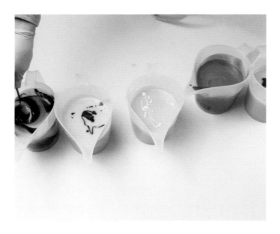

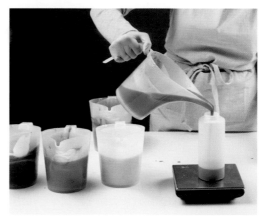

6 Divide the batter evenly among the five easy-pour containers (about 20 ounces/567 g in each). Add one dispersed color to each container and mix in by hand.

7 Pour 3 ounces (85 g) of each color into its own squirt bottle, making five squirt bottles, one of each color. Cap and set aside.

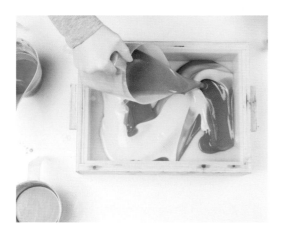

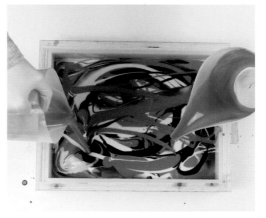

8 Pour from the easy-pour containers into the mold, using about a third of each color at a time in a random swirling pattern.

9 Alternate colors and the direction of your swirling motions until all the batter from the easy-pour containers is used.

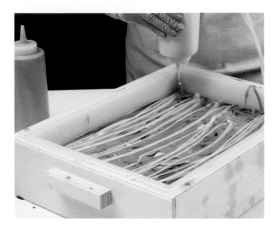

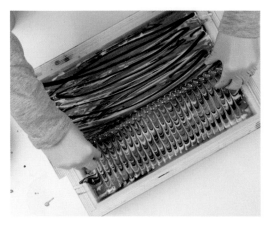

10 Squirt horizontal rows of color onto the swirled layers, again alternating colors until the bottles are empty. Make sure the rows in the top layer are neat and straight.

11 Insert the comb swirling tool along the long side of the mold into just the top striped layer of the soap batter. Slowly pull it straight across the surface, pulling it up and out when you reach the other side.

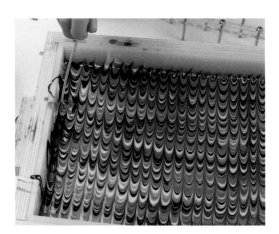

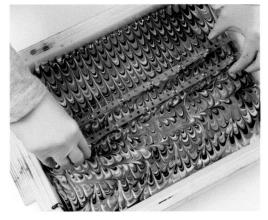

12 Use a chopstick if needed to make additional lines along the edges of the mold where the comb tool did not reach.

13 Insert the easy swirling tool into a corner of the mold, again just into the top layer. Pull the tool toward you while slowly moving it back and forth across the surface. Pull it up and out of the batter when you reach the other side.

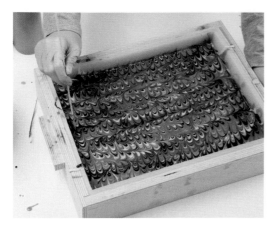

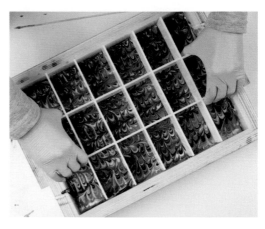

14 Use a chopstick if needed to touch up any swirls around the edges.

15 Insert the dividers into the mold.

Final Steps

Spray thoroughly with 99% rubbing alcohol several times over 90 minutes to prevent soda ash. Let sit at room temperature and wait at least 48 hours before unmolding.

Let the bars cure in a well-ventilated area for 4 to 6 weeks before using, turning them every few days to ensure they cure evenly.

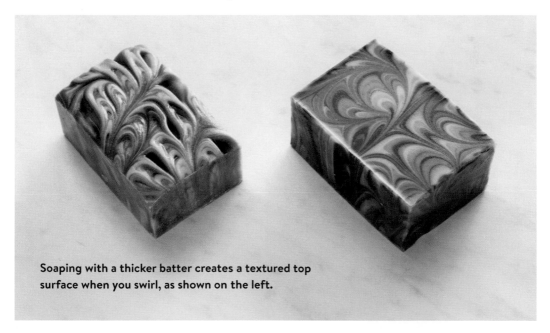

Soaping with a thicker batter creates a textured top surface when you swirl, as shown on the left.

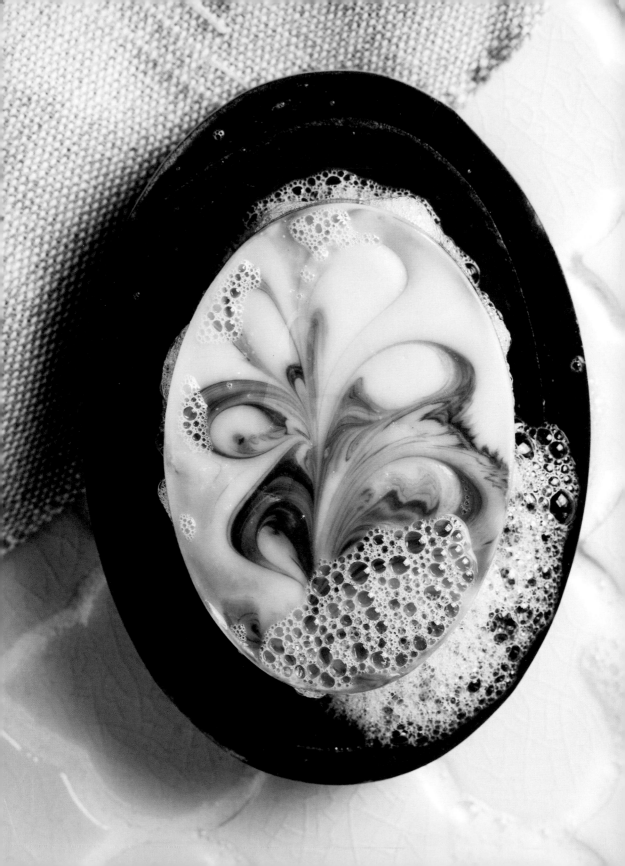

Coconut Milk In-the-Pot Swirl

with Kombucha

25% ADDED AT TRACE • MAKES 6 BARS

This recipe incorporates canned coconut milk and kombucha, both of which add extra sugar for lots of bubbly lather. An in-the-pot swirl creates a beautiful design that isn't hard to achieve, but the batter thickens quickly so be prepared to swirl!

Use unflavored kombucha so you're sure not to add anything unknown to the recipe. If you don't brew your own, there are many brands available with few additives.

Note that the bars go in the freezer overnight to prevent overheating.

Mold and Special Tools
6-bar oval silicone mold
Cutting board to move mold
　to freezer
2 easy-pour containers
Chopstick

Oil Amounts
4.0 ounces/113 g
　coconut oil (20%)
4.0 ounces/113 g
　palm oil (20%)
3.0 ounces/85 g
　rice bran oil (15%)
2.0 ounces/57 g
　cocoa butter (10%)
2.0 ounces/57 g
　hazelnut oil (10%)

2.0 ounces/57 g
　kukui nut oil (10%)
1.4 ounces/40 g
　sunflower seed oil (7%)
1.0 ounce/28 g
　shea oil (5%)
0.6 ounce/17 g
　castor oil (3%)

Lye-Water
3.4 ounces/96 g
　distilled water
2.7 ounces/68 g
　lye (4% superfat)
1½ teaspoons/7.5 mL
　sodium lactate

Fragrance Oil
1.4 ounces/40 g
　Tobacco and Bay Leaf

Essential Oil Alternative
1.9 ounces/54 g
　lime
0.5 ounce/14 g
　patchouli

Colorants
Disperse each into 1 table-spoon/15 mL hazelnut oil.

1 teaspoon/5 mL
　black oxide
1 teaspoon/5 mL
　green oxide

Additives
1.6 ounces/45 g
　canned coconut milk
1.6 ounces/45 g
　kombucha

Safe Soaping!

Wear proper safety gear the whole time · Work in a well-ventilated space · No distractions

Use Any Milk

As with all these recipes, you can substitute any other kind of milk or dairy product, used in the same amount.

Make the Soap Batter

1 Melt the palm oil in its original container, mix it thoroughly, and measure it into a heatproof bowl large enough to hold the entire recipe. Melt and measure the coconut oil and add it to the bowl. Add the cocoa butter to the hot oils and stir until melted. If needed, microwave the bowl in 10-second bursts to melt the butter completely. Add the hazelnut oil, kukui nut oil, rice bran oil, shea oil, sunflower seed oil, and castor oil and set the bowl aside.

2 Measure the distilled water and the lye into separate heatproof containers. Add the lye to the water a tablespoon (15 mL) at a time (never add the liquid to the lye). Stir continuously until the lye fully dissolves and the water becomes clear. Stir the sodium lactate into the lye-water.

3 When the oils and the lye-water have cooled to about 105°F (40.5°C), add the lye-water to the oils, pouring it over the shaft of the stick blender to minimize air bubbles.

4 Insert the stick blender into the batter, tilting it so that any trapped air can escape. *Do not turn on the stick blender until the blades are fully immersed.* Alternate pulsing and stirring with the stick blender until a thin trace is achieved.

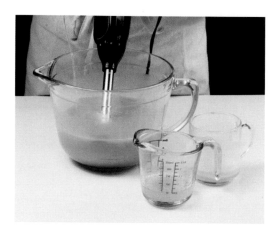

5 Add the fragrance oil, coconut milk, and kombucha and stick-blend until just incorporated.

Add a Little SCOBY

If you brew your own kombucha and would like to incorporate some of the benefits of the SCOBY into your soap, here's how: Reduce the amount of kombucha to 1.3 ounces (37 g) and add a small piece of SCOBY (0.3 ounce/8.5 g). Before adding the coconut milk and kombucha to the batter, grind the SCOBY into the mix with a mini blender, then continue with the recipe.

Color and Swirl

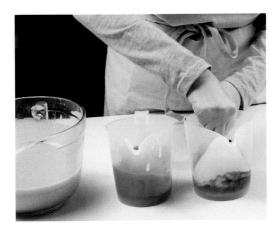

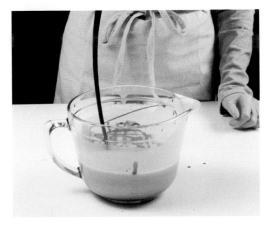

6 Pour about 2.5 ounces (71 g) of batter into the two easy-pour containers. Add ¼ teaspoon (1.2 mL) of dispersed black colorant to one and ¼ teaspoon (1.2 mL) of dispersed green colorant to the other. Mix well.

7 To make the swirl, pour each color, one at a time, into the uncolored batter. Pour them from higher up and in a circular motion so that the colored batter penetrates into and swirls throughout the uncolored batter.

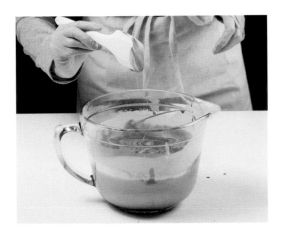

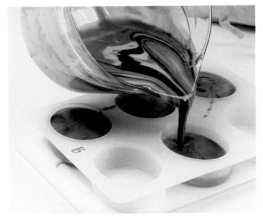

8 Stir the batter with a spatula, moving just once all the way around the bowl. Do not overmix.

9 Place the mold onto the cutting board for stability and pour the batter into the mold.

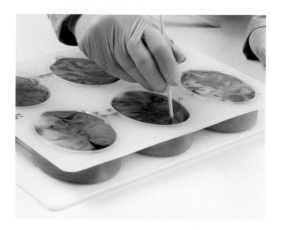

10 Swirl the tops with a chopstick inserted just under the surface of the batter.

Final Steps

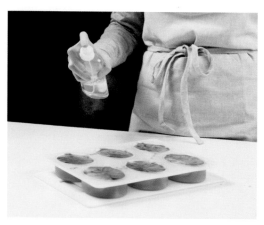

11 Spray thoroughly with 99% rubbing alcohol several times over 90 minutes to prevent soda ash. Place the mold in the freezer overnight to prevent overheating. Remove from the freezer and wait another 48 hours before unmolding. Frozen soaps tend to soften quite a bit as they thaw and need time to harden again.

12 Let the bars cure in a well-ventilated area for 4 to 6 weeks before using, turning them every few days to ensure they cure evenly.

Shimmied Layers
Castile Bars

50% ADDED AT TRACE • MAKES 10 BARS

This technique requires a steady hand — you will be pouring down the edges of the mold to create the stunning alternating petal-wave pattern. Because of the natural starches in rice milk, this recipe thickens more quickly than normal castile soap, so you need to start with a very thin trace to make the layers "shimmy" as they're meant to. Be prepared to pour fast!

Mold and Special Tools
Tall 12-inch (30.5 cm) silicone loaf mold
Chopstick
7 easy-pour containers
Soap beveller (optional)

Oil Amount
35 ounces/992 g pure olive oil (100%)

Lye-Water
5.7 ounces/161 g distilled water
4.5 ounces/128 g lye (4% superfat)
3 teaspoons/15 mL sodium lactate

Fragrance Oil Blend
1.3 ounces/37 g Lime
1.2 ounces/34 g Champagne

Essential Oil Alternative
0.8 ounce/23 g each bergamot, lemongrass, and grapefruit

Colorants
Disperse each into 1 table-spoon/15 mL pure olive oil.

1 teaspoon/5 mL Queen's Purple mica
1 teaspoon/5 mL Mermaid Blue mica
1 teaspoon/5 mL Kelly Green mica
1 teaspoon/5 mL Magenta mica

Natural Colorant Alternative
Container 1: ½ teaspoon/ 2.5 mL green oxide
Container 2: ¼ teaspoon/ 1.2 mL green oxide and ½ teaspoon/2.5 mL ultramarine blue pigment
Container 3: ½ teaspoon/ 2.5 mL ultramarine blue pigment
Container 4: 1 teaspoon/ 5 mL ultramarine violet pigment and ½ teaspoon/2.5 mL ultramarine blue pigment
Container 5: 1 teaspoon/ 5 mL ultramarine violet pigment
Container 6: ½ teaspoon/ 2.5 mL ultramarine violet pigment and ½ teaspoon/2.5 mL ultramarine pink pigment
Container 7: 1 teaspoon/ 5 mL ultramarine pink pigment

Additive
5.7 ounces/161 g rice milk

Safe Soaping!
Wear proper safety gear the whole time · Work in a well-ventilated space · No distractions

Use Any Milk
As with all these recipes, you can substitute any other kind of milk or dairy product, used in the same amount.

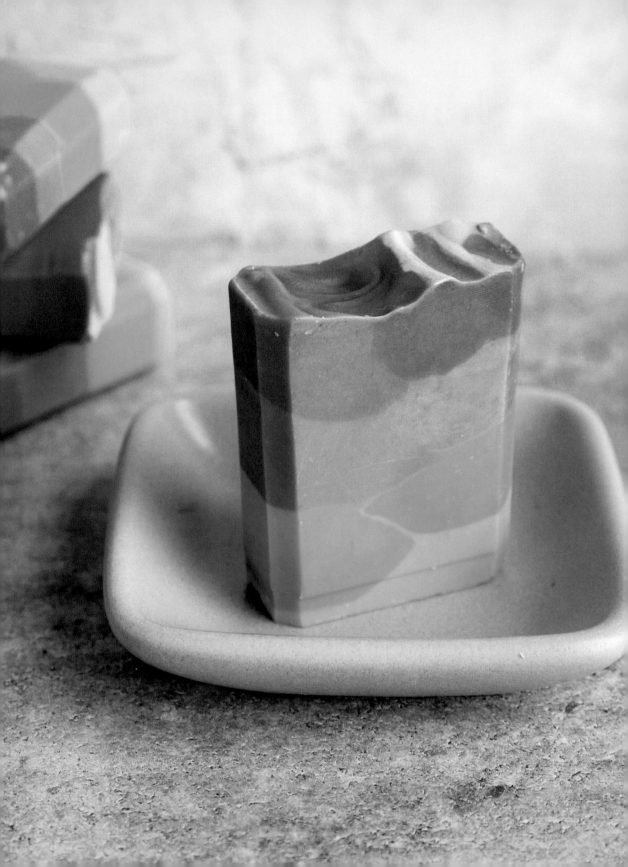

Prepare Ahead

Make the rice milk according to the instructions on page 10.

Make the Soap Batter

1 Measure the olive oil into a heatproof bowl large enough to hold the entire recipe. Heat the oil to 105°F (40.5°C) and set aside.

2 Measure the distilled water and the lye into separate heatproof containers. Add the lye to the water a tablespoon (15 mL) at a time (never add the liquid to the lye). Stir continuously until the lye fully dissolves and the water becomes clear. Stir the sodium lactate into the lye-water.

3 When the lye-water has cooled to about 105°F (40.5°C), add it to the oil, pouring it over the shaft of the stick blender to minimize air bubbles.

4 Insert the stick blender into the batter, tilting it so that any trapped air can escape. *Do not turn on the stick blender until the blades are fully immersed.* Alternate pulsing and stirring with the stick blender until a very thin trace is achieved.

5 Add the fragrance oil blend and rice milk. Stick-blend until combined, keeping trace thin.

Color and Pour

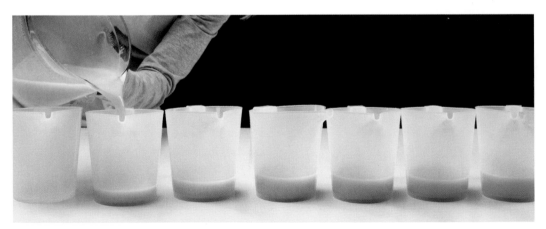

6 Divide the batter evenly among the easy-pour containers (about 7.5 ounces/ 213 g in each).

TECHNIQUE TIP
When dividing equal amounts of batter into a number of containers, measure the first amount on the scale and eyeball the remaining amounts.

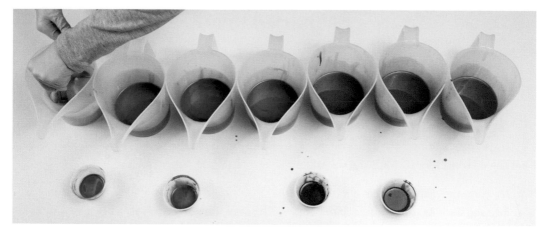

7   Add the colorants as follows:
- Container 1: 1 teaspoon (5 mL) dispersed Kelly Green
- Container 2: ½ teaspoon (2.5 mL) dispersed Kelly Green + ½ teaspoon (2.5 mL) dispersed Mermaid Blue
- Container 3: 1 teaspoon (5 mL) dispersed Mermaid Blue
- Container 4: 1 teaspoon (5 mL) dispersed Queen's Purple + ½ teaspoon (2.5 mL) dispersed Mermaid Blue
- Container 5: 1 teaspoon (5 mL) dispersed Queen's Purple
- Container 6: ½ teaspoon (2.5 mL) dispersed Queen's Purple + ½ teaspoon (2.5 mL) dispersed Magenta
- Container 7: 1 teaspoon (5 mL) dispersed Magenta

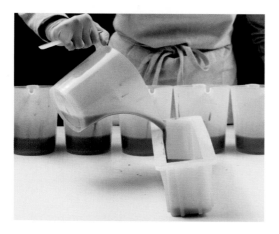

8   Prop the mold on a chopstick. Pour all of the plain green batter along the lower side of the mold so that it flows down the side and into the lower half of the mold. Do not pour straight into the mold.

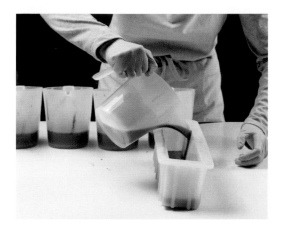

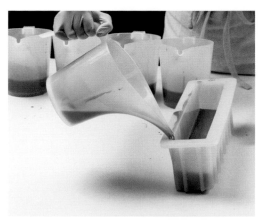

9 Move the chopstick to the other side of the mold and pour the green-blue batter on the opposite side of the mold.

10 Move the chopstick back to the other side of the mold. Gently scrape the batter from the previous pour into the soap, leaving a clean side to pour the plain blue batter.

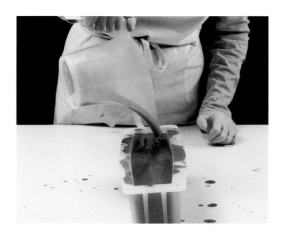

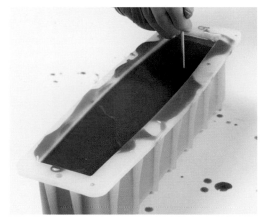

11 Continue moving the chopstick, scraping the sides of the mold, and pouring colors down the side in this order: purple-blue, purple, purple-magenta, and finally magenta. Remove the chopstick from under the mold and tap the mold gently if needed to even out the top.

12 Insert the chopstick into the very top of the soap; you are just swirling the top two colors. Make small circles down one long side of the mold, just to the middle of the batter.

Final Steps

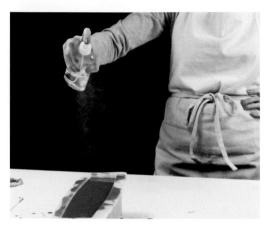

Spray thoroughly with 99% rubbing alcohol several times over 90 minutes to prevent soda ash. Let sit at room temperature for at least one full week before unmolding and slicing. Optional: bevel the edges of each bar to reveal even more of the design.

Let the bars cure in a well-ventilated area for 6 to 8 weeks before using, turning them every few days to ensure they cure evenly.

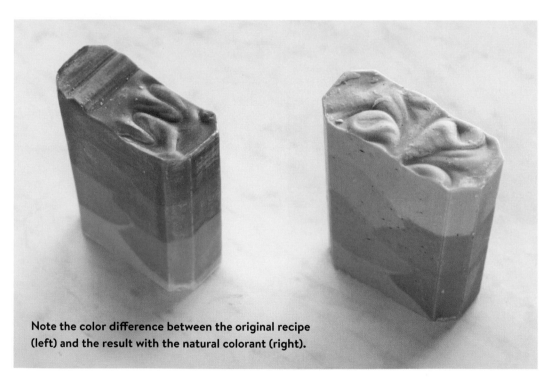

Note the color difference between the original recipe (left) and the result with the natural colorant (right).

Glossary

This is not a comprehensive guide to every term you will run into in your soapmaking journey, but it's a good start.

curing. Allowing the excess moisture in the bars to evaporate for 4 to 6 weeks, producing a gentler, harder, and longer-lasting bar. Castile soaps require a longer time to cure properly.

fixed oil. Also called fatty acid or carrier oil, a fixed oil is any oil of vegetable or animal origin that can be used to make soap or toiletries. Fixed oils may be liquid or solid at room temperature.

fragrance oil. A blend of aroma chemicals and essential oils synthesized specifically for a particular scent profile. While fragrance oils may contain natural elements, they are not considered all-natural ingredients.

gel phase. A phase during the soapmaking process in which saponification causes the soap to heat up and temporarily turn to gel. Gel phase can intensify colors in the soap and give it a shinier, slightly translucent look. However, not going through gel phase does not necessarily detract from a soap's quality. Some soapers prefer the matte look of ungelled soap and prevent gel phase by cooling the soap as quickly as possible. Many milk soaps are prevented from gelling to keep the milk from scorching.

lye discount (superfatting). A reduction in the amount of lye in a recipe, which leaves unsaponified oils in the finished soap for added skin-nourishing properties. The common discount (or superfatting) rate is between 3 and 10 percent.

SAP (saponification) value. The amount of lye needed for fixed oils to saponify, or become soap. This number varies based on the kind of fixed oil.

soda ash. A white, powdery film of sodium carbonate, a form of salt, that can form on soap when the lye and water react with carbon dioxide in the air instead of the fixed oils in the soap. It usually appears within the first 24 hours. It is not harmful, but it is unattractive.

sodium hydroxide. The alkaline used to saponify oils into soap. Potassium hydroxide is used to make liquid soap. Sodium hydroxide is also known as caustic soda or lye.

superfat. Excess oil in a recipe that does not saponify with lye, creating a soft, luxurious-feeling bar.

trace. The point at which a soap batter reaches emulsification. You can check for trace by pulling the stick blender out of the soap batter and dribbling batter back into the container; if the trails of batter remain visible for a few seconds, you've got trace! Trace ranges from light (a melted-milkshake consistency) to medium (a cake-batter consistency) to heavy (a pudding consistency). Trace progresses from thin to thick, and you cannot go backward. Once trace is achieved, you have just a couple minutes to pour the batter into the mold before the soap fully sets.

water discount. A reduction in the amount of liquid called for in a soap recipe (typically by 5 to 15 percent), which lessens drying time. The higher the water discount, the more likely the soapmaker will experience accelerated trace.

Frequently Asked Questions

Why do I need to use distilled water?
Tap water often contains minerals, metals, and other additives that can affect the outcome of the soap.

Why do I need to fully melt and stir the container of palm oil each time I use it?
Palm oil contains stearic acid, which settles in the bottom of the container. If you don't thoroughly mix the entire container before measuring, the bottom layer of unmelted oil will eventually contain a high percentage of stearic acid. Soap that contains too much stearic acid can be brittle and have white specks.

What can I add to increase lather?
Most commercially made soaps contain detergents to boost lather. These extra bubbles don't really get skin any cleaner, but consumers are now used to them and expect soap to have a lot more lather than handmade soaps typically provide. To increase lather, use coconut, palm, or castor oil; lower the superfat percentage to between 3 and 5 percent; or add sugar or honey at a ratio of 1 teaspoon per pound of oils.

Sugar can be dissolved in the lye-water, and honey can be warmed to melt any grains and added at trace. Keep in mind that adding sugar and honey to soaps can cause acceleration and will raise the temperature of the soap batter, so soap at cooler temperatures and place these soaps into the fridge or freezer to avoid overheating.

What is sodium lactate?
Sodium lactate is a salt derived from the natural fermentation of sugars found in corn and beets. Adding sodium lactate to the cooled lye-water helps the soaps harden more quickly so they can be unmolded faster. Harder bars also last longer! Sodium lactate is typically added at a ratio of 1 teaspoon per pound of oils. Adding too much can result in a brittle, crumbly bar of soap that may crackle in the mold.

How do I increase hardness in my bars?
Coconut oil, palm oil, babassu oil, palm kernel flakes, tallow, kokum butter, and cocoa butter all add hardness to soap. Other additives that do so include beeswax (at up to 8 percent), stearic acid (at 0.5 percent of your oils), sodium lactate (at 1 teaspoon per pound of oils), and various types of salts (which can be added straight to the batter or dissolved in the lye-water). Lowering the superfat to between 3 and 5 percent can also help.

Can I mix fragrance oils with essential oils?
Yes, as long as both are skin safe and you stay within the recommended usage rate for total amount of oils used.

Can I use materials like eye shadow, perfume, or crayon shavings to color and scent my soaps?
No. Finished toiletry items, makeups, or other products include many additional ingredients that are not suitable or safe for making cold-process soaps. These ingredients can

cause all sorts of problems in the batter, and they can morph and fade in the finished bars. They also may not be safe for use on the skin. All ingredients that go into soaps must be approved as skin safe.

Can I substitute the liquid in my recipe?

Yes. Substituting the liquid in a cold-process recipe can be done without needing to rerun the recipe through a lye calculator. Distilled water, milk, fruit purées, tea, wine, beer, floral waters, aloe vera, and many other liquids can be used in a soapmaking recipe. Research the liquid you want to use, as they all perform differently in soap and need to be prepared in specific ways. For example, tea will not color or scent the final soaps, alcohol needs to be boiled off before being used, and carbonated drinks must be opened and allowed to go flat.

Can I substitute or delete a recipe's oil or butter?

Yes, if you do so properly. Because different oils and butters require different amounts of lye to react with, when an oil or butter is changed in any way, the entire recipe must be rerun through a lye calculator to get a new lye amount. (See info on SAP values on page 16.) Also take into consideration the properties the original oil brings to the soap. Changing an oil, or completely removing one, can greatly affect the quality (lather, firmness, and so on) of the final bar.

Why do I need to measure by weight?

Measuring by weight is much more accurate than measuring by volume. It is always recommended for the oils, butters, lye, water, fragrancing agents, and most additives. One ounce of a heavy product like vitamin E oil has considerably less volume than one ounce of a lightweight oil like sweet almond oil. But some additives, such as exfoliants or colorants, are added by volume. Always follow the recommended measurement listed in the instructions.

Why do different soap calculators give different SAP values?

In cold-process soap, the saponification value (or SAP) represents the specific amount of sodium hydroxide required to bond with a specific amount of fats in order to become soap (that is, the amount of lye needed to safely turn the oils or butters into soap). Every oil and butter has a different SAP value. The exact SAP value for a specific oil or butter can vary slightly from crop to crop and season to season, so SAP values are usually a range of numbers rather than one specific number. That's why different soap calculators can give slightly different results.

How can I resize a batch to fit a different mold?

Soap calculators online usually have an option to resize recipes. Input the original recipe and then select "resize" to scale the recipe up or down. You will need to know how many ounces of soap the new mold can hold.

Why is my soap batter thickening so quickly?

Soap batter that thickens, or traces, quickly is said to have accelerated. Acceleration is most commonly caused by fragrance oils. Always check how a fragrance oil behaves before using it in your recipes. Soap batter can also thicken faster when you are soaping with lower temps and the hard oils or butters start to cool and solidify. This is often referred to as "false trace."

What are the small lumps in my soap batter?

Specks or lumps in batter are called "ricing." If the soap batter suddenly looks like tapioca pudding, it is due to the fragrance oils binding with hard oils in the soap. In some cases, the lumps can be stick-blended out, and the batter will get smooth again. However, this will significantly speed up trace and can result in a very thick batter that needs to be spooned into the mold rather than poured. To avoid ricing, purchase fragrance oils from reputable vendors that have fully tested their behavior in cold-process soap.

Why is my soap batter separating?

Separation can be caused by fragrance oils or failing to stick-blend long enough to reach true trace. It may look similar to ricing, but with separation there will be translucent swirls of oil throughout the batter. If the batter wasn't mixed long enough, the problem may be resolved by stick-blending. If it was caused by the fragrance oil, stick-blending may help, but you will most likely wind up with a very thick batter that may seize altogether.

Why did my soap batter suddenly turn solid (seize)?

When the batter starts to get gritty and thick like mashed potatoes while you're stick-blending, it's called "seizing." It's usually caused by fragrance oils that don't work in soapmaking. Seizing can also happen if you were trying to stick-blend out another problem, like ricing or separation.

What are the white bits (floaties) in my lye solution?

Lye (sodium hydroxide) typically contains a small amount of anticaking agent that does not affect the soapmaking process but can sometimes leave a residue in the lye solution. Undissolved lye will typically sink to the bottom of the liquid rather than rise to the top, so always stir the lye solution thoroughly and give it plenty of time to dissolve. If there are floaties in the lye solution, pour the solution through a fine-mesh strainer as you add it to the oils and butters.

How do I avoid air bubbles in my finished bars?

Air bubbles in finished bars look like white specks or small pockmarks. They are purely cosmetic. To avoid them, always pour the lye-water into the oils slowly and gently. Always stir gently when using whisks and spatulas. Tapping the mold on the work surface after you are finished pouring in the soap batter can also cause the air bubbles to rise up and out of the batter. This works best with thinner batter.

Why does my soap smell terrible when I first cut it into bars?

This issue is most common in milk soaps, but some fragrance oils will morph as the soaps air out. Always let your soaps cure four to six weeks before worrying too much about the scent.

What are the white/translucent lines and crackles in my soaps?

These are called glycerin rivers. Glycerin is a natural by-product of soapmaking. Glycerin rivers form when the glycerin gets too hot and begins to congeal in the soap. This is purely an aesthetic issue; the soaps are safe to use. To avoid glycerin rivers, fully disperse and mix the colorants well, lower the soaping temperatures, or use a water discount. If using titanium dioxide, micronize it with a coffee grinder or use at a lower rate.

Why is my soap soft and spongy?

If the soap has been in the mold for two or three days and/or has been allowed to sit out and cure for at least two weeks and is still very soft, it's unlikely to ever harden. Soft soaps can be caused by mismeasuring ingredients (not enough lye or too much oils), an improperly balanced recipe (too many soft oils and not enough hard oils or butters), or too much liquid in the recipe. These soaps are typically safe to use, but they will not last very long.

Why is my soap hard and brittle?

Soaps that are hard, brittle, or crumbly may contain too much lye. They are unsafe to use on skin and unfortunately can't be fixed, but depending on how much extra lye was added, they can sometimes be turned into a laundry soap. Check the pH of the soap to make sure. Soaps with too much sodium lactate (or other salt) can also be crumbly; these bars are safe to use but tend to fall apart.

Why did my soap crack down the middle?

This is usually caused by overheated soap, which can expand in the mold. This tends to happen with milk soaps, soaps with added sugars or honey, or soaps that were poured hot and then overinsulated. Less common reasons include too many hard butters, oils, wax, or salt in the recipe; too many dry ingredients (like clays) that absorbed the water out of the soap; or too much lye. Check the pH of the soap; if it isn't lye-heavy, the bars are fine to use.

What are the orange dots in my soaps?

"Dreaded orange spots" (commonly referred to as DOS) can appear while soap is still curing or they can show up months later. They are most commonly caused by rancid oils. Another cause of DOS can be using water that is not distilled. Superfatting too highly can also cause DOS, which is why most recipes are superfatted at 3 to 7 percent.

How long will my finished bars last?

Bars of cold-process soap don't have a specific expiration date, and some may last for many years. However, the shelf life can be affected by the oils that were used to make the soaps. If a high amount of an oil with a shorter shelf life was used, then the bars can develop DOS (see previous question), especially if the bars had a higher superfat amount. Soap with DOS is still safe to use but will look and smell unpleasant.

When soaping, you can add an antioxidant, such as grapefruit seed extract, rosemary oil extract, or vitamin E oil, to extend the shelf life of the oils and therefore the soaps.

Why is my soap melting so quickly in the shower?

Make sure to store soap that is being used in a soap dish that allows the water to drain out of the bottom. Soap left sitting in a pool of water will always become soft and squishy. Soaps that are formulated with a higher amount of liquid oils will be softer bars; these will dissolve faster than a bar with a harder formulation.

How long do basic soapmaking ingredients last?

Oils and butters all have different shelf lives; see chapter 3 for specific information.

Fragrance oils should be used within a year. After that the scents begin to morph and fade.

Essential oils have different shelf lives, but most will last at least a year before the scents start morphing and fading.

Micas and pigments last three to five years if kept dry and in the dark. Most other colorants last about a year.

Lye should be kept in a closed container in a dry space and used within a year. Expired lye is gray and may contain clumps.

How do I check the pH of my soap?

Testing the pH of finished soaps is always a good safety measure, especially if you suspect something may have gone wrong. Let the soap cure a few days, as freshly made soap can have a higher pH. To use a pH strips, create a lather with the bar and dip the testing end of the pH strip into the lather until it is fully saturated. Compare the color on the strip to the guide. A normal bar of handmade soap has a pH level of around 8 to 10.

A quick but less accurate method is the "zap" test. If you touch the tip of your tongue to the edge of the soap and feel a tingle (like licking a battery), then the soap is most likely lye-heavy.

Why is my lather colored?

If a soap bar is producing colored lather, too much colorant was used. While not dangerous, it often looks unpleasant and may stain washcloths and other items. There is no set rule on how much colorant to add, but we recommend dispersing 1 teaspoon (5 mL) of colorant into 1 tablespoon (15 mL) of a lightweight liquid oil, then adding the dispersion 1 teaspoon at a time to your batter until you get the color you like.

Resources

General Supplies

Bramble Berry
360-734-8278
www.brambleberry.com

From Nature with Love
800-520-2060
www.fromnaturewithlove.com

Frontier Co-op
844-550-6200
www.frontiercoop.com

GloryBee
800-456-7923
https://glorybee.com

Hoegger Supply Company
770-703-3072
https://hoeggerfarmyard.com

Liberty Natural Products
800-289-8427
www.libertynatural.com

Majestic Mountain Sage
435-755-0863
https://www.thesage.com

Mountain Rose Herbs
800-879-3337
https://www
.mountainroseherbs.com

San Francisco Herb Co.
800-227-4530
www.sfherb.com

SoapEquipment.com
765-530-0307
https://soapequipment.com

Summers Past Farms
619-390-1523
https://www.
summerspastfarms.com

Wild Weeds
707-839-4101
www.wildweeds.com

Essential Oils, Fragrance Oils, and Colorants

Rainbow Meadow, Inc.
800-207-4047
https://www.rainbowmeadow
.com

Soapgoods
https://www.soapgoods.com

Wholesale Supplies Plus
800-359-0944
www.wholesalesuppliesplus.com

Oils and Fats

Oils of Aloha
800-367-6010
https://oilsofaloha.com

Soaper's Choice
833-257-6627
https://soaperschoice.com

Spectrum Chemical Manufacturing Corp.
800-772-8786
https://www
.spectrumchemical.com

Welch, Holme & Clark Co., Inc.
973-465-1200
https://www.whc-oils.com

Tutorials

Soap Queen
Bramble Berry
www.soapqueen.com

Cultures for Yogurt, Kefir, Sour Cream, and Buttermilk

New England Cheesemaking Supply Co.
413-397-2012
https://cheesemaking.com

Cultures for Health
https://www
.culturesforhealth.com

Index

ACKNOWLEDGMENTS

I could never do the creative work I do without the support of a dedicated team at home. My family experiments with me, laughs with me at the (many) failures, and then helps me clean up the mess.

The Bramble Berry team is the most dedicated, kind, and creative group of people anyone could ever hope to work with. Special thanks to Nicole P. for keeping all the recipes organized, testing some super-out-of-the-box ingredients, and helping me stick to a writing schedule in the midst of small-business, working-mom chaos.

Finally, the soapers and creative artisans who cheer me on @bramble-berry and @comemakewithme on Instagram inspire me every single day, and for that I am grateful.

Expand Your Soapmaking Horizons
with More Books by Anne-Marie Faiola

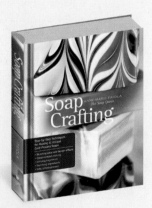

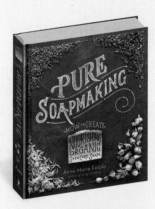

Making soap is easy! This one-stop resource for soapmakers of all skill levels includes 31 recipes and step-by-step instructions. Explore the full range of special effects, colors, additives, and molds available.

Make luscious, nourishing soaps with a palette of all-natural ingredients such as coconut butter, almond oil, coffee grounds, green tea, and more. Step-by-step photography guides you through every stage of cold-process soapmaking.

Join the conversation. Share your experience with this book, learn more about Storey Publishing's authors, and read original essays and book excerpts at storey.com.
Look for our books wherever quality books are sold or call 800-441-5700.